Airman and Family Resilience

Lessons from the Scientific Literature

Sarah O. Meadows, Laura L. Miller, Sean Robson

RAND Project AIR FORCE

Prepared for the United States Air Force
Approved for public release; distribution unlimited

T0308359

For more information on this publication, visit www.rand.org/t/RR106

Library of Congress Cataloging-in-Publication Data is available for this publication.

ISBN: 978-0-8330-9075-1

Published by the RAND Corporation, Santa Monica, Calif.

© Copyright 2015 RAND Corporation

RAND® is a registered trademark.

Support RAND

Make a tax-deductible charitable contribution at
www.rand.org/giving/contribute

www.rand.org

Preface

This report documents research and recommendations that RAND offered to the Air Force to help strengthen the development of a new office responsible for resilience and to promote Airman and family resilience. U.S. military personnel have been engaged in operations in Central Asia and the Middle East for the past decade. Many aspects of deployments have the potential to contribute to individual stress, such as uncertainty about deployment dates and lengths; fear of or confrontation with death or physical injury; separation from friends and family members; and reintegration after deployment. Service members and their families also manage other military-related stressors, such as frequent relocations, long work hours, and family separations. Some service members and their families may cope well or even thrive as they overcome adversity and accomplish challenging tasks. However, some may suffer negative consequences as a result of military-related stressors, such as physical injury; depression, anxiety, or other mood disorders; post-traumatic stress disorder; substance abuse; family dysfunction; and, in extreme cases, even suicide or suicide attempts. With the aim of preventing such deleterious outcomes, rather than simply responding to them, the study of resilience is of paramount importance.

This study is the final overarching report in a series of nine that resulted from that research effort. It provides an introduction to resilience concepts and research and highlights findings from domain-specific literature reviews. It also documents the recommendations that RAND provided to the Air Force to address its desire to track the resiliency of Air Force personnel and their families and to develop organizational resilience initiatives across the Air Force.

The goal of the larger RAND project was to assist the Air Force in understanding how to assess and track the total fitness of the force and develop programs to increase the resiliency of military and civilian Air Force personnel and their families. At the time of the project, staff members assigned to the new Air Force Resilience Office were not subject matter experts and lacked the time to research and assess the literature themselves. They wanted to ensure that their efforts were not just based on popular claims and general notions but that they aligned with current science. Thus, they asked RAND researchers to provide clear, concise reviews of the eight Total Force Fitness (TFF) domains: medical, nutritional, environmental, physical, social, spiritual, behavioral, and psychological.

Eight supplemental, companion reports outline the constructs, metrics, and influential factors relevant to resiliency across those eight domains of TFF. These reports are not intended to be a comprehensive review of all literature within a domain. Rather, they focus on studies that consider the stress-buffering aspects of each domain, regardless of whether the term *resilience* is specifically used. They also include a review of the literature supporting a direct association between key factors in each domain and well-being. This expanded the reviews' scope to include a broader range of applicable studies and also allowed for terminology differences that occur across different disciplines (e.g., stress management, hardiness). The results of our studies may help broaden the scope of research on resilience and help Airmen and their families achieve optimal fitness.

The research reported here was sponsored by the Air Force offices of Airman and Family Services (AF/A1S), the Surgeon General (AF/SG), and the Secretary of the Air Force, Force Management and Personnel (SAF/MRM) and conducted within the Manpower, Personnel, and Training Program of RAND Project AIR FORCE.

RAND Project AIR FORCE

RAND Project AIR FORCE (PAF), a division of the RAND Corporation, is the U.S. Air Force's federally funded research and development center for studies and analyses. PAF provides the Air Force with independent analyses of policy alternatives affecting the development, employment, combat readiness, and support of current and future air, space, and cyber forces. Research is conducted in four programs: Force Modernization and Employment; Manpower, Personnel, and Training; Resource Management; and Strategy and Doctrine. The research reported here was prepared under contract FA7014-06-C-0001.

Additional information about PAF is available on our website:
http://www.rand.org/paf

Table of Contents

Figures

Tables

Summary

In recent years, the U.S. military has increasingly focused on how service personnel and their families respond to an array of stressors related to demanding deployments across the nation and around the world, including more than a decade of combat operations in Central Asia and Iraq. Deployment has the potential to contribute to individual stress, with such factors as uncertainty about assignment time lines; culture shock in theater; fear of or confrontation with death or physical injury; environmental challenges, such as extreme climates and geographical features; austere living conditions; separation from friends and family members; and reintegration after deployment. Service members and their families also manage other military-related stressors, such as frequent relocations, long work hours, and the additional family separations associated with unaccompanied tours and domestic training exercises. Individuals and families may cope well or even thrive as they overcome adversity and accomplish challenging tasks. But some may suffer negative consequences as a result of military-related stressors, such as physical injury, including traumatic brain injury; depression, anxiety, or other mood disorders; post-traumatic stress disorder; spiritual crises; substance abuse; family dysfunction; marital problems and dissolutions; social isolation; and, in extreme cases, even suicide or suicide attempts. Top military officials have expressed alarm at the increasing suicide rates in the ranks and, in considering the demands and hardship on service personnel and their families, have committed to ensuring that they receive the support they need. With the aim of preventing rather than simply responding to deleterious outcomes, the study of resilience has taken on paramount importance to military leaders, especially in the Air Force.

In fiscal year 2011, the Air Force offices of Airman and Family Services (AF/A1S), the Surgeon General (AF/SG), and the Secretary of the Air Force, Force Management and Personnel (SAF/MRM) asked RAND to conduct a literature review. The goal was to assist the Air Force in understanding how to assess and track the total fitness of the force and develop programs to increase the resiliency of military and civilian Air Force personnel and their families. The staff members assigned to the new Air Force Resilience Office to lead efforts on this new issue were not subject matter experts and lacked the time to research and assess the literature themselves. They wanted to ensure that their efforts were not just based on popular claims and general notions but that they aligned with current science.

They asked that RAND researchers also adopt and adapt to what the U.S. armed forces already had outlined as the concept of Total Force Fitness, with service personnel and families who are "healthy, ready, and resilient; capable of meeting challenges and surviving threats" (Mullen, 2010, p. 1) This notion of "fitness" is directly related to the concept of resilience, and TFF reflected the collective effort of scholars, health professionals, and military personnel, who outlined what they saw as its eight domains: medical, nutritional, environmental, physical, social, spiritual, behavioral, and psychological.

This overarching report builds on the foundation of the eight previous studies—all designed to be succinct and accessible to the nonspecialist—on each of those domains. It brings together highlights of the reviews and documents their relevance to Air Force metrics and programs. This report provides a more in-depth introduction to resilience concepts and research, presents a RAND model of the relationship between resilience and TFF, and documents Air Force resiliency efforts and metrics for tracking the resiliency of Air Force personnel and their families at the time of this study. The research identified the following key themes:

- Resilience can be studied only in the context of stress.
- It is a process, rather than a static set of traits or characteristics.
- Individuals do not have a static, set amount of resilience or resilience resources or factors.
- Key resilience resources/factors broadly include personality factors, behaviors, external resources, and biology/physiology.

By comparing information found in the research literature to Air Force practices and data collection at the time, this study also provided seven recommendations aimed at supporting the development of initiatives to bolster resilience across the Air Force, including the following:

- Promote regular unit physical activity and hold commanders accountable for the physical fitness of their military personnel.
- Better resource Health and Wellness Centers to increase capacity for targeted interventions by subject matter experts.
- Continue to leverage Wingman Day[1].
- Add a Programs and Services tab to the Air Force Base website template.
- Increase sharing of resilience-related data across the Air Staff.
- Fill gaps in data collection.
- Strengthen the ability of the Air Force Resilience Office (which preceded the Comprehensive Airman Fitness Office) to promote resilience factors across the force.

The research also underscored that there is no survey instrument, professional assessment, or biological test available today with which commanders can determine who in their unit will or will not be resilient in the face of stress. Predicting human behavior is extremely difficult. In social science, the best predictors tend to capture only a small percentage of the variance. Resilience is in a constant state of fluctuation; resilience resources and stressors can come and

---

[1] Wingman Day is a program that helps Airmen and their families cope with stress and builds on the concept of Airmen taking care of Airmen (i.e., Airmen acting as "wingmen"). Typically a Wingman Day will consist of day-long activities, including team-building exercises and group learning sessions, designed to build comradery and a sense of group identity. Topics vary from year to year and installation to installation but generally highlight ways in which Airmen and their families can maintain and strengthen elements of Total Force Fitness (discussed later in this report).

go. But the literature can help the Air Force build individual and community capacity to be resilient by understanding which factors shape the experience and interpretation of stressors, responses to stressors, and associated changes to well-being and resilience resources, if any, following the event.

Acknowledgments

This research was sponsored by the Air Force Resilience Office and was led by Mr. Brian P. Borda for a significant portion of the study period and by then Air Force Surgeon General Lt Gen (Dr.) Charles B. Green, and Mr. William H. Booth, then Deputy Assistant Secretary of the Air Force for Force Management Integration (SAF/MRM).

We would like to thank the action officers from the sponsoring offices for their role in shaping the research agenda and providing feedback on interim and final briefings of the research findings. Those officers are Maj Kirby Bowling, our primary contact from the Air Force Resilience Office; Col John Forbes and Lt Col David Dickey from the Air Force Surgeon General's office; and Ms. Linda Stephens-Jones from SAF/MRM. We also appreciate the insights and recommendations received from Ms. Eliza Nesmith while she was in the Air Force Services office and from Lt Col Shawn Campbell while he served in the SAF/MRM office.

This manuscript benefited from the editorial skills of Craig Matsuda and Patricia Bedrosian. Arwen Bicknell improved the appearance and readability of the tables in the appendix. We also thank Kirsten Keller for her feedback on an earlier version of this report and our two reviewers, Dawne Vogt and Megan Beckett.

Abbreviations

AF/A1S	Air Force Airman and Family Services
AF/SG	Air Force Surgeon General
ARS	Adolescent Resiliency Scale
BEST	Biographical Evaluation and Screen of Troops
BMT	basic military training
BPFI	Baruth Protective Factors Inventory
BRCS	Brief Resilient Coping Scale
BRS	Brief Resiliency Scale
CAIB	Community Action Information Board
CD-RISC	Connor-Davidson Resilience Scale
CHAMP	Consortium for Health and Military Performance
CMS	ClassMaps Survey
COR	conservation of resources
DCoE	Defense Centers of Excellence for Psychological Health and Traumatic Brain Injury
DECA-C	Devereux Early Childhood Assessment Clinical Form
DoD	Department of Defense
DRRI	Deployment Risk and Resilience Inventory
DRS	Dispositional Resilience Scale
DUI	driving under the influence
ER-89	Ego Resilience Scale
HAWC	Health and Wellness Center
HIPAA	Health Insurance Portability and Accountability Act
HWP	health and wellness program
LBQ	Lackland Behavioral Questionnaire
MHS	Military Hardiness Scale
MRT	master resilience training
PAF	Project AIR FORCE
PBS	Perceived Benefits Scale
PPE	personal protective equipment
PRP	Penn Resiliency Program
PTG	post-traumatic growth

PTGI	Post-Traumatic Growth Inventory
PTGI-C	Post-Traumatic Growth Inventory for Children
PTSD	post-traumatic stress disorder
PVS-III-R	Personal Views Survey III-R
RASP	Resiliency Attitudes and Scales Profiles
RBS	Resilience as a Belief System
RS	Resilience Scale
RSA	Resilience Scale for Adults
RSCA	Resiliency Scales for Adolescents
RSES	Response to Stressful Experiences Scale
SAF/MRM	Secretary of the Air Force, Force Management and Personnel
SMS	Short Message Service
SOC	Sense of Coherence
TBI	Traumatic Brain Injury
TFF	Total Force Fitness
TRS	Trauma Resilience Scale
USAF	United States Air Force

1. The U.S. Military, Resilience, and Total Force Fitness

U.S. military personnel have been engaged in operations in Central Asia and the Middle East for the past decade. Members of the armed forces also deploy to other regions of the world. Many aspects of deployments have the potential to contribute to individual stress, such as uncertainty about deployment time lines; culture shock in theater; fear of or confrontation with death or physical injury; environmental challenges, such as extreme climates and geographical features; austere living conditions; separation from friends and family members; and reintegration after deployment. Service members and their families also manage other military-related stressors, such as frequent relocations, long work hours, and the additional family separations associated with unaccompanied tours and domestic training exercises. Some service members and their families may cope well or even thrive as they overcome adversity and accomplish challenging tasks. However, some may suffer negative consequences as a result of military-related stressors, such as physical injury, including traumatic brain injury; depression, anxiety, or other mood disorders; post-traumatic stress disorder (PTSD); spiritual crises; substance abuse; family dysfunction; marital problems and dissolutions; social isolation; and, in extreme cases, even suicide or suicide attempts (Tanielian and Jaycox, 2008; Ramchand et al., 2011). With the aim of preventing rather than simply responding to such deleterious outcomes, the study of resilience is of paramount importance.

This RAND Project AIR FORCE (PAF) report represents the overarching synthesis of a series of eight reports on resiliency. All nine reports adopt the Air Force definition of resilience: "the ability to withstand, recover and/or grow in the face of stressors and changing demands," which, as this report will show, encompasses a range of definitions of resilience represented throughout the scientific literature. By focusing on resilience, the armed forces aimed to expand their care to ensure the well-being of military personnel and their families through preventive measures and not just by treating members after they begin to experience negative outcomes (e.g., depression, anxiety, insomnia, substance abuse, PTSD, or suicidal ideation). Below, we provide the necessary background for this report including a brief description of resilience research in the military, define the related concept of Total Force Fitness (TFF), define the objective of this resilience study, and point out some possible limitations of our approach.

Suicide Prevention and Military Interest in Resilience Research

In the 20th century, scientific interest in resilience tended to focus on attempts to understand why some children raised in poverty or under great adversity grew up to live successful lives whereas others struggled mentally, physically, or economically (Simmons and Yoder, 2013). However, after such events as the September 11th attacks, large natural disasters, such as Hurricane Katrina, and military operations in Iraq and Afghanistan, U.S. researchers began to focus on resilience following traumatic events in adulthood (Simmons and Yoder, 2013).

For the military, continuous stressful operating conditions have become a valuable setting not only in which to study resilience but also to apply existing knowledge. Many service members and their families can deal with problems in their lives; some even thrive because they survive demanding experiences. However, the military's focus on resilience seeks to reduce the number of those who cannot cope effectively and those whose mental and physical well-being suffers as a result of stress and strain.

The U.S. military's large-scale interest in resilience can be traced to leaders' alarm at the suicide rate among U.S. service members—deaths occurring despite concerted efforts to (1) educate the force about suicide risk, (2) identify at-risk individuals, (3) increase access to mental health care, and (4) reduce the stigma that attaches to those who seek help. In 2008, the reported suicide rate was highest in the Marine Corps and the Army (19.5 and 18.5 suicides per 100,000, respectively), followed by the Air Force and the Navy (12.1 and 11.6 suicides per 100,000, respectively) (Ramchand et al., 2011, p. xiv). The Army's suicide rates hit a 28-year high in 2008 (Kuehn, 2009), and Army leaders looked to the concept of resilience for a fresh approach to the problem (Simmons and Yoder, 2013). Army Chief of Staff General George W. Casey, Jr., turned to the founder of positive psychology, Martin Seligman, and his Penn Resiliency Program (PRP) for insights (Seligman, 2011).[2] Ultimately, General Casey invested $145 million for the PRP to develop the Global Assessment Tool as a test for soldier resilience and psychological health, basic and advanced online resilience-related instruction for soldiers following the test, and an in-person master resilience training (MRT) program for noncommissioned officers (Seligman, 2011). General Rhonda Cornum became director of this new Comprehensive Soldier Fitness program (now Comprehensive Soldier and Family Fitness and discussed further in Chapter 2), and her own career served as a public example of the resilience ideal. As a major, Cornum served as a flight surgeon in the 1991 Persian Gulf War, where she survived a helicopter crash, multiple injuries (including broken arms that

---

[2] Other major Army efforts at this point included a five-year $50 million agreement with the National Institute of Mental Health for a prospective study of suicidal thoughts and actions among soldiers (Kuehn, 2009).

her captors left untreated for days), and more than a week as a prisoner of war (Cornum and Copeland, 1993). The Army's attention to resilience placed a spotlight on resilience scholarship that drew the other services' attention as well.

The Department of Defense Concept of Total Force Fitness

At this time, DoD more broadly was also taking steps to adopt and apply aspects of positive psychology and resilience research. In 2009, Admiral Michael Mullen, Chairman of the Joint Chiefs of Staff (JCS) from 2007 to 2011, asked the Consortium for Health and Military Performance (CHAMP) at the Uniformed Services University of the Health Sciences to develop a comprehensive Total Force Fitness (TFF) concept. Admiral Mullen outlined the TFF concept in a special issue of the journal *Military Medicine*: "A total force that has achieved total fitness is healthy, ready, and resilient; capable of meeting challenges and surviving threats" (Mullen, 2010, p. 1). Thus, this notion of "fitness" is directly related to the concept of resilience. Together with the Samueli Institute, the Institute of Alternate Futures, and members of the JCS, CHAMP hosted a workshop with over 70 experts to define what the military should focus on to keep its personnel resilient and flourishing within that operating environment. Out of that workshop emerged working groups, members of which authored journal articles that were subjected to the scientific peer review process. The ultimate product of that effort, the special issue of *Military Medicine,* reflected the collective effort of scholars, health professionals, and military personnel who drew on the research literature to outline what they saw as eight domains of TFF. These domains, shown in Figure 1.1 are medical, nutritional, environmental, physical, social, spiritual, behavioral, and psychological.

The first four domains, shown in blue, were described as elements of fitness of the body; the latter four, shown in dark green, are described as elements of fitness of the mind. This framework expanded the traditional conceptualization of resilience by looking beyond the psychological to also emphasize the mind-body connection and the interdependence of each of the eight domains. Note that the idea of total fitness applies to collectivities as well as individuals, hence the term total *force* fitness. Fitness, then, is relevant to active duty and reserve and guard Airmen, civilian Airmen, as well as their families. Ultimately, TFF is integral to the Air Force because it sets that stage for readiness.

Figure 1.1. DoD's Eight Domains of Total Force Fitness Are Interdependent

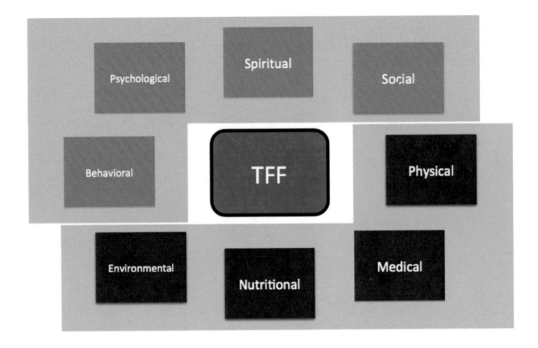

Study Objectives

In fiscal year 2011, the Air Force offices of Airman and Family Services (AF/A1S), the Surgeon General (AF/SG), and the Secretary of the Air Force, Force Management and Personnel (SAF/MRM) asked RAND to conduct a literature review on resilience using the special issue of *Military Medicine* as a point of departure. The goal was to help the Air Force understand how to assess and track the total fitness of the force and develop programs to increase the resiliency of military and civilian Air Force personnel and their families. The staff members assigned to the new Air Force Resilience Office to lead efforts on this new issue were not subject matter experts and did not have the time to research and assess the literature themselves. They wanted to ensure that their efforts were not just based on popular claims and general notions but that they aligned with current science.

Although the Air Force organizes its resilience efforts around the simpler four-domain scheme (mental, physical, social, and spiritual) that existed before TFF was developed, the research sponsors requested that RAND adopt the eight TFF domains as the organizing framework for the literature review. The eight domains of total force fitness can easily be integrated into the Air Force's four-domain typology, so modifying the typology is not necessary to encompass the concepts. The spiritual and social pillars match directly. The Air Force's physical pillar then would comprise the TFF's physical, environmental, medical, and nutritional domains. The Air Force's mental pillar would include the TFF's psychological and behavioral domains. We acknowledge that all domains contain "behaviors," although, because the original conceptualization of TFF treats health behaviors as a separate, distinct domain, we have chosen to do the same.

We followed the general framework spelled out in the special issue of *Military Medicine*, although in some cases we adapted the scope of a domain to better reflect relevant research we identified. Thus, this study resulted already in eight reports, each focusing on resilience-related research on constructs, measures, and interventions to promote fitness within one TFF domain (McGene, 2013; Robson, 2013, 2014; Shih, Meadows, and Martin, 2013; Yeung and Martin, 2013; Flórez, Shih, and Martin, 2014; Robson and Salcedo, 2014; Shih et al., 2015). However, we note that these domains are not all mutually exclusive. For example, the spiritual and social domains overlap when members' religious communities provide a source of social support. The reports were designed to provide high-level overviews of the literature accessible to the nonexpert rather than long, highly technical reviews aimed at an expert, academic audience.

This overarching report builds on the foundation of eight previous reports on each domain. It brings together highlights of each review and documents the reports' relevance to Air Force metrics and programs. For the full reviews, including bibliographies, we refer readers to those reports. This report provides an in-depth introduction to resilience concepts and research, presents our model of the relationship between resilience and TFF, and documents Air Force resiliency efforts and metrics for tracking the resiliency of Air Force personnel and their families at the time of this study. By comparing information we found in the research literature to Air Force practices and data collection at the time, we could provide recommendations aimed at supporting the development of initiatives to promote resilience across the Air Force.

This report reflects resiliency concepts and Air Force–specific recommendations provided to the Air Force at the conclusion of the study along with the initial domain-specific literature reviews. However, since that time, the RAND team has authored the eight domain-specific reports and those reports have undergone scrutiny from subject matter experts in those fields. No two reports were reviewed by the same set of reviewers, and additional research was incorporated as a result of that process. Thus, because this report was published last, it benefitted from questions about the resiliency concept that arose during those previous reviews and is able to reflect the final framing of those other literature reviews.

Study Approach and Limitations

Air Force leaders are interested in promoting resilience among active and reserve component Airmen, civilian employees, and Air Force family members. The research sponsors requested that RAND identify resilience-related constructs and measures in the scientific literature and report any evidence of initiatives that promote resilience across a number of domains. We did not limit our search to research conducted in military settings or with military personnel[3]; Air Force leaders sought the potential opportunity to apply results of these studies to a population not yet addressed (i.e., Airmen). Further, many Air Force services support Air Force civilians and family members. Thus, results of civilian studies would apply to these populations.

We also reviewed the types of resilience-related measures collected by the Air Force. However, it was not feasible for us to collect, synthesize, and analyze the actual data to try to create a resilience profile for different subpopulations in the Air Force community. Evaluation of the effectiveness of Air Force programs, services, or initiatives was also beyond this project's scope.

Organization of This Report

Chapter 2 explores the concept of resilience, including how scholars have defined and attempted to measure it, nonmilitary programs designed to promote it, and how it relates to the TFF concept. Chapter 3 provides a brief summary of each of the eight TFF domains: medical, nutritional, environmental, physical, social, spiritual, behavioral, and psychological. This chapter summarizes results from the TFF domain reports and provides key take-aways about important resilience factors that contribute to health and well-being. It also offers a review of interventions, programs, and policies that aim to increase the well-being in each domain. Interested readers are encouraged to refer to these individual reports for more detailed information on the TFF domains. Chapter 4 characterizes resilience-related data currently available to the Air Force. Finally, Chapter 5 offers recommendations for the Air Force to continue promoting resilience among Airmen, their families, and civilian employees. An appendix contains a table of measures developed to assess resilience and related constructs (e.g., hardiness, flourishing, and

---

[3] It is worth noting that, relative to studies on civilians, there are fewer family resilience studies specifically focused on *military families* and even fewer that are Air Force–specific. Both are reasons for our broad search strategy.

post-traumatic growth [PTG]) among both adults and children/adolescents, along with notes about their focus, reliability, validity, and source.

2. Understanding Resilience

> "It is not the strongest of the species that survive, nor the most
> intelligent, but the one most responsive to change."
>
> — Charles Darwin

This chapter explores the concept of resilience, including how scholars have defined it, how it has been measured, how nonmilitary programs are designed to promote it, and, finally, how it relates to the TFF concept. The Air Force sponsors of this research wanted to ensure that the Air Force definition aligned with that in the research literature, and their efforts were grounded in a scientific understanding of the relationship between resilience factors, stress, and well-being.

Defining Resilience

Theories of resilience have been influenced by multiple disciplines. The most prominent resilience theories grew out of child development and psychopathology research and sought to explain why some children who experienced trauma in early childhood showed mental health problems whereas others did not. Subsequent theories have been generated in subareas within psychology, including clinical and positive psychology, as well as such disciplines as sociology, biology, nursing, and medicine.

Regardless of discipline, *resilience* is generally defined as the ability of an individual to "bounce back" after experiencing stress, although there is no single, universally accepted definition (Wald et al., 2006; see Meredith et al., 2011 for a review of resilience definitions). This definition assumes that stress negatively affects well-being and that individuals can do things or access resources to counteract that negative effect. How individuals use resilience resources generally is referred to as *coping*. We refer to individual attributes, characteristics, qualities, and environmental factors that provide a foundation for resilience as *resilience resources;* these are sometimes called *resilience factors* in the literature.

Related terms often are used in the general resilience literature, and it is important to understand their similarity to and differences from the concept of resilience. Hardiness refers to a personality type that promotes resilience—characterized by control, commitment, and challenge—that can handle stress and strain effectively and not let it lead to negative outcomes (Kobasa, 1979; Kobasa and Maddi, 1977; Bartone et al., 1989). Sense of coherence (SOC), focused on the way people perceive and respond to

9

events in their lives, is defined by three components: comprehensibility, manageability, and meaningfulness (Antonovsky, 1993; Antonovsky and Sagy, 1986). Flourishing extends the "bounce back" in the definition of resilience to functioning at even higher levels and experiencing ever greater levels of well-being than before the stress occurred (Keyes, 2002). Flourishing is sometimes referred to as thriving (Carver, 1998; O'Leary and Ickovics, 1995) or post-traumatic growth (Tedeschi and Calhoun, 2004). It is also worth noting that the severity and intensity of the experienced stress required for PTG to occur generally are very high. It is perhaps unsurprising, then, that most of this literature is relevant to individuals who experience trauma (e.g., childhood abuse, a violent crime, combat) rather than stress. Of these related constructs, hardiness and SOC have been studied extensively in relation to stress (Eriksson and Lindström, 2006; Eschleman, Bowling, and Alarcon, 2010). Despite these constructs' different origins, there is considerable overlap in theory and subsequent predictions for health and well-being (Almedom, 2005). The components of these multidimensional constructs are discussed in later chapters (i.e., psychological fitness, spiritual fitness, social fitness).

Air Force Definition of Resilience

The Air Force has adopted the Defense Centers of Excellence for Psychological Health and Traumatic Brain Injury (DCoE) definition of resilience. As noted in the previous chapter, resilience is "The ability to withstand, recover and/or grow in the face of stressors and changing demands" (Defense Centers of Excellence, 2011).[4] This definition highlights three aspects of resilience. First, the definition refers to resilience as an *ability,* suggesting that it does not come as a stable, unchanging quantity. Despite certain genetic predispositions, individuals are not born with a set and unchanging ability to handle stress. It is important to note that some aspects of resilience, or some resilience resources or resilience factors, are easier than others to change or develop. Hardiness, generally thought of as a personality trait, typically is not viewed as being as flexible as physical activity level, which an individual can more easily change. More recent research suggests that hardiness is malleable (Maddi et al., 2009; Judkins et al., 2006; Zach et al., 2007) but not to the degree of other resilience factors. Second, the DCoE definition of resilience encompasses elements of both resilience and flourishing by allowing for not just recovering following stressors but also for *growth.* By emphasizing *withstanding*

---

[4] There is some debate in the literature about exactly what patterns of resilience look like. For example, some researchers suggest that resilience requires that an individual function as well after stress as before, whereas others allow for the notion of a "new normal" level of functioning. Although detailed discussion of this debate is beyond the scope of the current study, interested readers should consult the work of Bonanno (2005) for a discussion of resilience trajectories.

stress, the definition also includes elements of hardiness. Thus, the DCoE definition of resilience is consistent with other definitions found in the literature, and it broadly combines elements of hardiness, resilience, and flourishing. And third, the DCoE definition focuses on *changing demands,* suggesting that resilience is a process that occurs over time.

A Note About Stress

Inherent in the definition of resilience is the notion of *stress.* The bounce back definition assumes that stress has a negative effect on well-being and that individuals can do things or access resources to counteract that negative effect. Stress can be episodic, or a single event, or it can be chronic and occur over time. For Airmen and their families, stress can occur at any time—in peacetime, in wartime, before a deployment, during a deployment, or after a deployment. Often, service members endure repeated stressors that do not affect typical civilian families, testing their ability to be resilient in the face of stress, strain, and trauma. These include frequent deployments, separation, and relocations, all of which are hallmarks of military life and can have a significant effect on the family (Jensen, Lewis, and Xenakis, 1986; Segal, 1986). Military spouses routinely report that deployments are the most stressful aspect of military life (Rosen and Durand, 2000). Further, within the deployed environment, Airmen can face uncertainty about deployment time lines; culture shock in theater; fear of or confrontation with death or physical injury; repeated exposure to traumatic combat situations; environmental challenges, such as extreme climates and geographical features; austere living conditions; and missing key family milestones at home (e.g., birthdays, holidays). And reintegration after deployment is also seen as a particularly stressful time, by both service members and family members, especially spouses (Sayers, 2011). McEwen and Stellar (1993) coined the term *allostatic load* to refer to the wear and tear on the body that occurs as a result of repeated exposure to episodic or chronic stress. Although originally applied to the physiological effect of stress, it is not difficult to imagine a similar psychological effect of stress. As we discuss more below, stress eats away at the resources that individuals have, and use, to combat stress.

Research Approaches to Resilience

In academia, how researchers think about a problem progresses as more knowledge is generated. Richardson (2002) outlined three major approaches to resilience that appear in the literature, and they are important to understand because they shape how resilience theories influence resilience research. Richardson says different lines of research ask *what* makes people resilient, *how* people are resilient, and *why* people are resilient. Despite an implied chronology, these approaches overlap in their influence on resilience research.

The first major approach to resilience research focused on traits and qualities either present or absent within an individual.[5] This emphasis grew out of a literature that moved from emphasizing risk factors associated with negative well-being outcomes to a view that emphasized protective factors that prevent negative outcomes from occurring. A potential pitfall of this approach, which treats resilience as a set of individual traits and qualities, is that it implies that the ability to be resilient is finite and does not change. This notion of stability is especially problematic for developmental psychologists for whom change over time is an integral part of their doctrine (see Rutter, 1985, 2007).

The second major approach to resilience, unsurprisingly, shifted attention away from static traits and qualities to how people both acquire and use resilience resources (Rutter, 1987). This line of research focuses on how people manage their problems and is more in line with the idea that resilience is a process. This approach generally is credited with introducing the idea that resilience is not just about recovering from stress to reach some state of equilibrium but that it also should include the notion of growth. Research in positive psychology best exemplifies this approach (Seligman and Csikszentmihalyi, 2000).

Richardson (2002) describes a third approach that treats resilience as an internal drive to self-actualize. This approach sees resilience as not about how resilient people behave, think, or feel, or what qualities, skills, or resources resilient people possess, but rather as about what drives people to be resilient in the first place. It focuses not on whether individuals want to be resilient but assumes that they do and seeks to uncover what drives or motivates them to be just that. Richardson describes resilience in this approach as a "force." He notes that this may be the oldest approach to resilience, despite its postmodern feel.

Our own approach focuses on resilience resources or resilience factors that can be fostered through systematic efforts to promote resilience. The general construct of resilience is amorphous and similar in this way to health or well-being. From a research and policy perspective, nothing in the definition alerts us as to what to do to make someone more resilient. What are the qualities and characteristics that make someone resilient? What actions do resilient individuals take and how do they behave? An approach that focuses on resilience factors gives us a place to focus our research and

---

[5] Although the earliest examples of this approach viewed resilience factors as "all or nothing," more recent formulations take the view that individuals have varying *levels* of traits and qualities associated with resilience.

policy efforts. Our approach mixes elements of the three approaches outlined by Richardson (2002): traits and qualities, actions and behaviors, and motivations to be resilient.

Critiques of Resilience Research

Despite the increased popularity of resilience research and a corresponding increase in its volume, a number of critiques have appeared in the literature. First, although many theories of resilience are intuitively appealing, not all are empirically derived, and often, few empirical tests of theories exist. Second, although resilience generally is thought of as a process, many theories and their corresponding tests, are described in the cross-section. That is, few studies use longitudinal data to follow the same individuals over time as they cope with stress; such data are needed to confirm the underlying processes of resilience suggested by these theories. And third, concepts within resilience theories are not always well defined, making problematic the measurement of resilience's key components. Nonetheless, several measures currently exist that purport to measure resilience and related constructs, which we discuss in the section below.

Measurement of Resilience

Many scales, most often derived from self-report survey data, seek to measure resilience and related constructs (e.g., hardiness, flourishing, and PTG) among adults, children and adolescents. The appendix contains a table of measures that we have collected, including a description of and information about the psychometric properties and source of each scale. Generally, these measures contain 20 to 50 self-rated items that have demonstrated acceptable psychometric properties. They exhibit high internal consistency, suggesting that the items tend to measure the same construct or subconstructs, and high construct validity, suggesting that they are actually measuring the ability to cope with stress (e.g., the scales are associated with the outcomes of resilience, such as positive mental health, as one would expect). As an example, the Connor-Davidson Resilience Scale (CD-RISC) comprises 25 items that are self-rated on a five-point scale ranging from "rarely true" to "true nearly all the time" (Connor and Davidson, 2003). Example items include "See the humorous side of things" and "Not easily discouraged by failure." The scale reflects five general factors: (1) "personal competence, high standards, and tenacity," (2) "trust in one's instincts, tolerance of negative affect," (3) "positive acceptance of change, and secure relationships," (4) "control," and (5) "spiritual influences" (Connor and Davidson, 2003, p. 80).

There are some limitations in the applicability of these measures. First, few have been extensively evaluated in the research literature, although there are exceptions (e.g., the CD-RISC and the Resilience Scale (RS) [Wagnild and Young, 1993]). Consequently, "it is not yet clear what resilience questionnaires actually measure" (Bonanno, Westphal, and Mancini, 2011, p. 18). Because resilience typically is the domain of psychologists, who tend to use college students as respondents, many measures have been used or validated only or primarily among student samples. College students clearly are not representative of the average population.

Second, for this report's purposes, it is important to note that most of these measures have not been used with military populations. There are a few exceptions, including the Military Hardiness Scale (Dolan and Adler, 2006), the Deployment Risk and Resilience Inventory (DRRI) (King et al., 2006), and the Response to Stressful Experiences Scale (RSES) (Johnson et al., 2011). These scales were constructed specifically for use with service members and accordingly focus mostly on military demands, combat-related trauma, and stress. Although the scales were developed only recently, positive results have been found in the few studies using them. The Military Hardiness Scale has been used in studies demonstrating that hardiness buffers against deployment stressors (Dolan and Adler, 2006) and is positively associated with psychological well-being (Skomorovsky and Sudom, 2011). The DRRI has been associated with both mental and physical health measures (Fikretoglu et al., 2006; Vogt et al., 2008).

And third, it is unclear whether these resilience measures can be used to assess a resilience program's effect. If a measure treats resilience as a snapshot rather than as a process over time, then it may not be sensitive to changes in resilience resources that programs target. Thus, if research uses pre- and postintervention measures of resilience to assess whether a policy change, program, or other type of intervention has an effect, and that measure cannot detect behaviors and psychological and social resources that are used to cope with stress, then research may mischaracterize the effectiveness of interventions. Further, if a change is detected pre- and postintervention, many existing resilience measures cannot determine which factors changed within the individual to produce that change.

Programs to Develop Resilience

Attempts to teach resilience largely have focused on children and adolescents. Indeed, the PRP, one of the most extensively studied programs to prevent depression, targeted an age range from 10 to 14 (Brunwasser, Gillham, and Kim, 2009). Meta-analyses, which use statistical analyses to aggregate results across a number of individual, stand-alone studies, generally find small to moderate (versus large) effects[6] for programs targeting prevention of depressive symptoms in children and adolescents (Brunwasser, Gillham, and Kim, 2009; Horowitz and Garber, 2006; Stice et al., 2009), suggesting that although these programs do, on average, have some preventive or salubrious effect on mental health, they are not able to completely mitigate symptoms. Although the PRP was developed initially for children and adolescents, the Army has modified its content for integration into MRT as part of the Comprehensive Soldier Fitness program.[7] This training is designed to "increase core competencies in optimism, mental agility, self-regulation, self-awareness, self-efficacy, and connection" (Meredith et al., 2011, p. 145). Because this program is relatively new and has not been subjected to independent and objective evaluation, evidence of its effectiveness is not yet available (Smith, 2013; Steenkamp, Nash, and Litz, 2013). However, the Army program's evaluation of its own implementation found that self-reported resilience and psychological health (measured along four fitness domains: emotional, family, social, and spiritual) was more desirable in Brigade Combat Teams with MRT than in units without; 18- to 24-year-olds in MRT units were especially likely to score higher on those measures (Lester et al., 2011). The program has both supporters and critics whose assertions have yet to be rigorously assessed. Critics posit that some combat veterans may experience the program's promotion of positive emotions and optimism as dismissing or minimizing their negative emotions, and thus the program could contribute to feelings of self-condemnation and shame, limiting their ability to work through painful feelings of guilt and remorse and to successfully reintegrate (Smith, 2013).

Other programs promoting resilience have been developed for adults and the working population. Williams LifeSkills® has demonstrated effectiveness in reducing both psychosocial and cardiovascular stress indices (Bishop et al., 2005; Davidson et al., 2007; Gidron, Davidson, and Bata, 1999; Kirby et al., , 2006; Williams et al., 2009). The program targets individuals with psychosocial risk factors associated with such chronic disease as coronary heart disease. Such risk factors considered by the program include depression, work stress, low socioeconomic status, and social support. This training program focuses on ten skills designed to "reduce negative psychosocial factors like hostility/anger, depression, anxiety and perceived stress, and to increase positive factors like self-esteem, optimism, and satisfaction with life" (Williams and Williams, 2011, p.

---

[6] To help compare effect sizes, we provide an example comparing a large effect size to a small effect size. A large effect size of .8 means that the average individual in the treatment group would score better (e.g., on a measure of depression) than 79 percent of individuals in a control group receiving no treatment. A small effect size of .2 means that the average individual in the treatment group would score better than 58 percent of individuals in the control group.

[7] The Air Force has since adopted MRT as part of its Comprehensive Airman Fitness program.

304). In general, these skills emphasize awareness, problem solving, and interpersonal transactions.

HardiTraining®, another example of a commercial resilience training program, is "based on a workbook that includes hardy coping, socially supportive interactions, and self-care exercises, plus a procedure for using the feedback from these efforts to deepen hardy attitudes" (Maddi, 2007, p. 67). This program was developed to target the general population more broadly (e.g., working adults) to help develop and promote hardy attitudes and actions. However, the program has also been promoted to help in the rehabilitation of returning military personnel who have experienced physical or mental trauma.

This type of training was found to be effective in increasing self-reported hardiness and social support while decreasing self-reported strain and illness severity (Maddi, Kahn, and Maddi, 1998). However, others have found that a more intensive one-day course also may provide some immediate changes in hardiness, but these benefits largely dissipate over time (Tierney and Lavelle, 1997). Although some empirical evidence has been provided to support these and other commercially driven programs, additional research is needed to demonstrate that training results in long-term changes in resilience and well-being.

Relationship Between Resilience and Total Force Fitness

Although it may appear that resilience and TFF are distinct concepts, we argue that, in fact, what we call *resilience factors* simply are key constructs within TFF domains. We show this relationship between resilience factors and TFF in Figure 2.1. Four aspects of this model should be highlighted.

First, the model depicts a process, rather than a static, snapshot. On the left of the figure, at stage 1, an individual has a prestress capacity to deal with stress and strain. These prestress resources can be thought of as resilience factors. Thus, we operationalize the capacity to be resilient as the resource pool an individual has within and across the eight TFF domains. In Chapter 3, we review the key resilience factors across the eight domains but provide an example here. Having a strong support network at stage 1 could be considered a resilience factor in the social domain. These are not mutually exclusive domains: They all function together. An individual may lack fitness in one domain but still be resilient overall because of all of the other resilience factors available to draw on.

Figure 2.1. The Relationship Between Resilience Factors, Total Force Fitness, and Stress

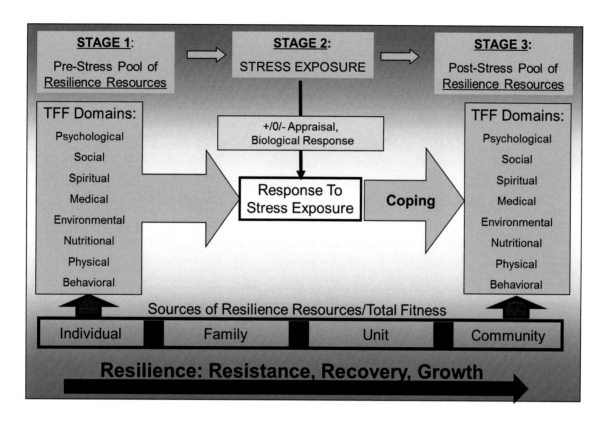

Second, at the bottom of the figure, resilience capacity can be a function of factors available at the individual, family, unit, and community levels (as indicated by the arrow pointing to the box at the bottom of the figure to the stage 1 prestress pool of resilience resources). For example, some resilience factors, such as coping style, are at the individual level, whereas social support can be garnered from the family, unit, or community level. An Airman's unit could provide informational support (e.g., how to use certain protective gear). And, a religious community could provide a different type of support. These are depicted as the foundation on which this process occurs. Certain stressful events may require use of resilience factors at only one level (e.g., individual); others may require that an individual tap into available resources at multiple levels. The key to successful coping is that individuals have an arsenal of available resilience resources and factors at multiple levels.

Third, an individual's appraisal of a stressful event or chronic strain determines if, and how, resilience factors are mobilized. At stage 2 in our model, an individual encounters some type of stress, strain, or trauma, then determines whether it is a threat

17

(i.e., negative [-]), neutral [0], or in some cases, positive [+].[8] Stress, it should be noted, elicits a biological response in the body, even if an individual is not consciously aware of it (Brierley-Bowers et al., 2011; Chrousos, 1998). If, through cognitive appraisal, the stress is determined to be negative, individuals can use their resilience factors (or prestress capacity) to cope with stress. In Figure 2.1, this is represented in a blue arrow labeled "Coping" between stages 2 and 3. Alternatively, if the stress is not perceived as negative, individuals may not have a stress response, not tap in resilience capacity, and pass directly through stage 2, into stage 3.[9]

At stage 3, the individual has confronted the stress (or not), used resources (or not), and changed behaviors (or not). How well the individual managed stress can once again be measured by total fitness, or the resource pool available to the individual across the eight TFF domains. For example, someone who has successfully handled it should not have developed mental or physical symptoms as a result of that stress (such as chronic worrying, insomnia, pain, and fatigue) and not have adopted maladaptive coping strategies (withdrawing from social interaction, overeating, or abusing drugs or alcohol). Lack of fitness at this stage is an indicator that the individual could not manage stress and may not be able to cope with more of it in the future. At this point in the process, it is appropriate to assess whether an individual has (or has not) resisted, recovered, or grown as a result of exposure to stress. That is, the trajectory from stage 1 to stage 2 to stage 3 is what we would call resilience. This is denoted by the black arrow at the bottom of the figure.

Fourth, the stages in the model can overlap: At any given moment, an individual may be preparing simultaneously for stress yet to come (stage 1), appraising an existing stressor (stage 2), and managing an existing stressor (stage 3). To assert that an individual's strong social network is evidence of his or her capacity for resilience, it also is necessary to observe that an individual has experienced stress.

The U.S. Navy and Marine Corps (Department of the Navy, 2010) use the metaphor of "leaky buckets" to express the stress and resilience process (see Figure 2.2). To describe this metaphor briefly, leaks represent stressors and chronic strains that drain personal resources essential to overall well-being. In fact, conservation of resources

---

[8] Positive stress is called *eustress* in the literature (Selye, 1978) and examples of it may include being promoted at work, getting married, or having a child.

[9] Compared to the original biological stress response model proposed by Selye (1950), which suggested that all stress evoked the same physiological and biological response, more recent research suggests that cognitive appraisals can shape physiological responses to stress (Kemeny, 2003). Thus, whether an individual views a stressful situation as controllable or not has different implications for the body's physiological response.

Figure 2.2. The Leaky Bucket Metaphor for Stress

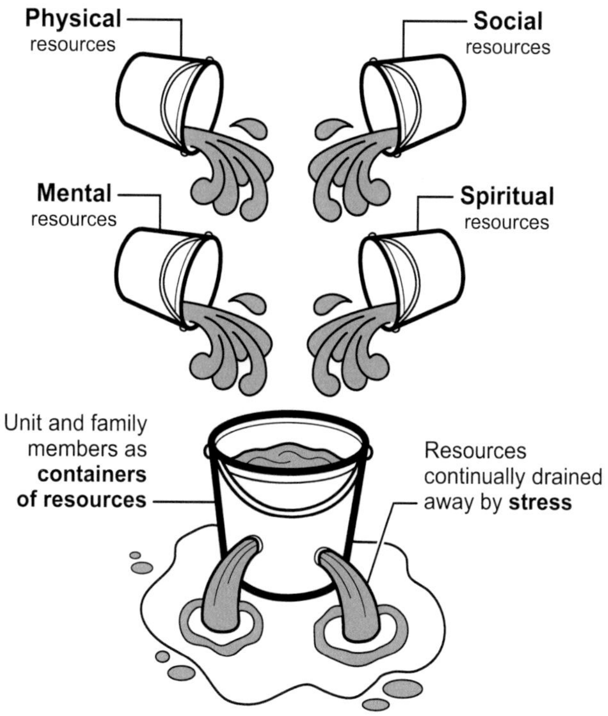

Physical resources · Social resources · Mental resources · Spiritual resources · Unit and family members as **containers of resources** · Resources continually drained away by **stress**

SOURCE: Adapted from the Department of the Navy (2010).

(COR) theory suggests that the extent to which such leaks or stressors have drained important resources for coping with stress is a strong predictor of response to trauma (Hobfoll, 1989, 2011). Although efforts should be made to modify or eliminate stressors, this is not always possible, especially in a military environment. Consequently, an important principle of COR is to promote and restore individual personal resources that promote well-being and recovery when the individual experiences a stressful or traumatic event.

Thus, "[t]he 'leaky bucket' analogy highlights the two targets for reducing the negative consequences of stress—minimizing or eliminating stressors to slow the depletion of available resources and storing up and replenishing resources that have been depleted by stress" (Department of the Navy, 2010, p. 3-2). As noted above, repeated exposure to episodic or chronic stress is detrimental to the pool of resilience resources available to an individual and can thus make it more difficult to be resilient in the face of stress. This metaphor of the leaky bucket is particularly relevant to our resilience research as we attempt to identify ways to identify the personal resources available to an individual and interventions and strategies to promote, replenish, and build these.

Main Versus Buffering Effects of Resilience Factors

Two types of associations exist between resilience factors and well-being outcomes: main and buffering. The model we present in Figure 2.1 allows for either main or buffering effects of resilience resources: Resilience factors across the eight domains of TFF can be related to individuals' well-being, independent of whether they experience a stressor, or those same factors can be used to cope in the presence of a stress.

Figure 2.3 depicts a main effect of a resilience factor (shown by the blue line). In this case, the resilience factor has an effect on mental health, but this association does not depend on whether a stressor is present (see Pearlin et al., 1981). Experiencing a stressor also has an independent, direct effect on well-being (shown by the black line). In this model, it is not necessary to know whether an individual has experienced a stressor to assess whether the resilience factor has an effect on well-being.

Compare the main effect depicted in Figure 2.3 to the buffering effect depicted in Figure 2.4. In a buffering effect, resilience factors have an association with well-being only in that they counteract the negative effect of stress on well-being. Thus, resilience resources influence well-being only in the presence of stress (shown by the blue line) (Pearlin et al., 1981; Wheaton, 1985). Thus, resilience resources *buffer* stress. In this model, as in the main effect model, stress has a direct association with well-being (shown by the black line). In this model, it is necessary to know whether an individual has experienced a stressor to assess whether resilience and resilience factors have an effect on well-being; resilience can be understood only in the context of stress.

Figure 2.3. Main Effect of Resilience on Well-Being

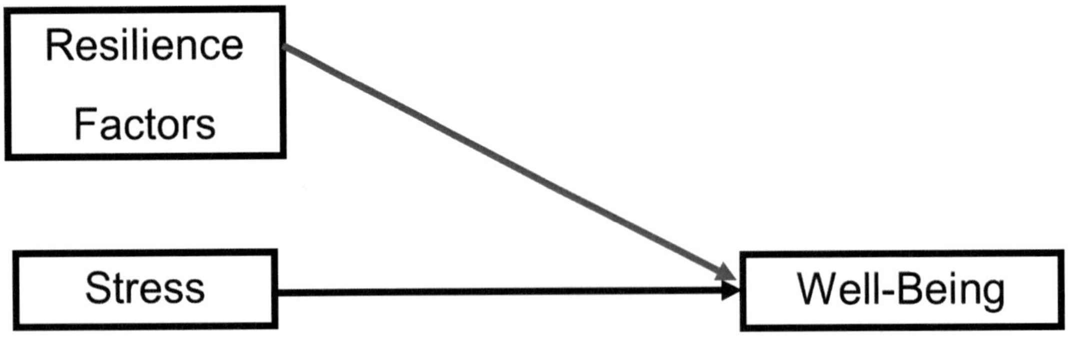

Figure 2.4. Buffering Effect of Resilience on Mental Health

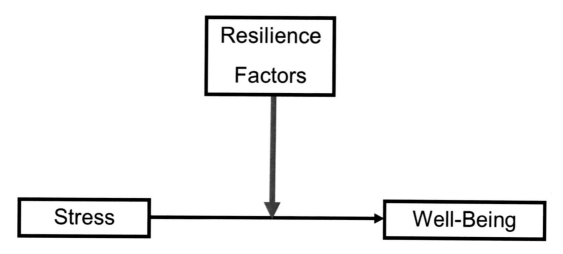

To provide an example, consider the role of social support from a spouse in predicting overall mental health. In the main effect model, spousal social support is independently, positively associated with mental health. It is unnecessary for a spouse to experience a stressful life event or chronic strain to feel the salubrious effects of receiving a partner's emotional support. But in the buffering model, a spouse would see positive effects of a supportive partner only if he or she also experienced stress. If stress is absent, then social support is not useful. Obviously, resilience resources most likely have *both* a direct *and* a buffering effect on well-being. Most resilience resources can directly enhance well-being and contribute to an individual's overall fitness level *and* can be used to combat stress or strain when it occurs. The important thing to remember is that, unlike fitness, *resilience* cannot be observed outside stress's presence; response to it is part of resilience's definition.

Summary

To summarize, our review of the general resilience literature identified key themes. First, resilience can be studied only in the context of stress. If you take a snapshot of someone's well-being at a given point in time, lack of negative outcomes may simply signal the absence of stress. Similarly, evidence of having sufficient resilience resources or resilience factors can be observed only in stress's presence. It is important to note that science has identified which resilience resources/factors will be most useful to most people under most stressful conditions. A review of the general resilience literature can identify key constructs within the eight TFF domains that are directly associated with overall well-being and those that are associated with well-being by buffering stress.

Second, resilience is a process, rather than a static set of traits or characteristics. Individuals may be resilient in one context but not another. And how an individual behaviorally, cognitively, and emotionally responds to stress can vary considerably from stressor to stressor. This variation implies that coping and responding to stressful situations, threats, and daily problems is a process that evolves as contexts change.

Third, individuals do not have a static, set amount of resilience or resilience resources/factors; resilience is not completely defined by early life experiences; and resilience is not a dichotomy or an either/or quantity. Over time, individuals can develop a larger repertoire of resilience resources and resilience factors, although chronic stress and trauma can also erode these, particularly when individuals employ unhealthy coping strategies.

Fourth, key resilience resources/factors broadly include personality factors, behaviors, external resources, and biology/physiology (Masten and Obradovic, 2006; Polk, 1997). Throughout the rest of the report, we highlight important resilience resources and resilience factors that fall within these broad categories, organizing them into the eight TFF domains.

Finally, a number of existing measures purport to assess resilience and related constructs among both adults and children and adolescents. No single measure is preferred over others, few have been used in military populations, and fewer still have been used to assess the effectiveness of programs that aim to increase or improve individual resilience. Similarly, existing programs designed to positively affect resilience have limitations that make it uncertain as to whether they achieve their intended effects.

3. Resilience-Related Scientific Research In Each of the Total Force Fitness Domains

> "I have heard there are troubles of more than one kind.
> Some come from ahead and some come from behind.
> But I've bought a big bat. I'm all ready you see.
> Now my troubles are going to have troubles with me!"
>
> — Dr. Seuss

We have briefly reviewed the general literature on resilience, thus far, and how it is operationalized and measured. In much of this literature, although not all, the term *resilience* is most often used as a synonym for well-being or psychological health. However, resilience is by definition linked to the experience of stress. Without stress, there can be no resilience. The same is not true of general well-being or psychological health. But what the Air Force/DCoE definition of resilience cannot tell us is how to make an Airman, family member, or civilian more resilient. This makes the definition difficult to apply from a research and policy perspective.

Thus, we recommended that the Air Force focus on the importance of resilience factors and their association with well-being. High (and low) levels of resilience resources can result in more (or less) ability to cope with stress and strain. In some instances, these resilience factors are directly associated with well-being. In others, these factors come into play when an individual faces a stressful event or chronic strain. In this case, resilience factors have a buffering effect on well-being and an effect on reducing stress' negative consequences. It is this buffering effect of resilience factors that we can label resilience.

We also linked the concept of TFF to resilience via resilience factors (Mullen, 2010). To recapitulate, the eight domains of TFF are medical, nutritional, environmental, physical, social, spiritual, behavioral, and psychological. The resilience factors in these domains provide an arsenal of resources that individuals can use to combat stress. Or, said another way, resilience resources are Dr. Seuss's "big bat." In the eight other reports in this series, we defined for each domain what it means to be fit, identified key resilience factors, noted the state of each line of research in measuring those factors, reviewed the literature linking them to well-being and other relevant outcomes, and, finally, offered insights into interventions aimed at increasing overall domain fitness as well as into factors associated with domain fitness. Below, we briefly summarize the key points from each of the TFF domain reports.

RAND Project AIR FORCE Series on Resiliency

The research sponsors requested that RAND adopt the eight TFF domains as the organizing framework for our literature review. We followed this general framework outlined in the special 2010 issue of *Military Medicine* described in Chapter 1, although in some cases we adapted the scope of a domain to better reflect the relevant research.[10] Thus, this study resulted in eight peer-reviewed reports, each focusing on resilience-related research in one TFF domain, of which we note that not all are mutually exclusive. These eight reports define each domain and address the following interrelated topics:

- medical: preventive care, presence and management of injuries, chronic conditions, and barriers and bridges to accessing appropriate quality health care (Shih, Meadows, and Martin, 2013)
- nutritional: food intake, dietary patterns and behavior, and the food environment (Flórez, Shih, and Martin, 2014)
- environmental: environmental stressors and potential workplace injuries and preventive and protective factors (Shih et al., 2015)
- physical: physical activity and fitness (Robson, 2013)
- social: social fitness and social support from family, friends, coworkers/unit members, neighbors, and cyber communities (McGene, 2013)
- spiritual: spiritual worldview, personal religious or spiritual practices and rituals, support from a spiritual community, and spiritual coping (Yeung and Martin, 2013)
- behavioral: health behaviors related to sleep and to drug, alcohol, and tobacco use (Robson and Salcedo, 2014)
- psychological: self-regulation, positive and negative affect, perceived control, self-efficacy, self-esteem, optimism, adaptability, self-awareness, and emotional intelligence (Robson, 2014).

These reports are not intended to be comprehensive reviews of all the literature in a domain. Rather, they focus on studies that consider stress-buffering aspects of each domain, regardless of whether the term *resilience* is specified. They also include a review of the literature supporting a direct association between key factors in each domain and well-being. This expanded the reviews' scope to include a broader range of studies and allowed for differences in terminology used across different disciplines (e.g., stress management, hardiness). Our primary goal was to identify evidence of interactive effects (i.e., those that buffer the negative effects of stress), but as noted above, we did not exclude research evidence supporting direct effects (i.e., those that promote general well-being).

---

[10] For example, the social fitness domain was extended beyond the primary focus on group cohesion featured in the *Military Medicine* article by Coulter, Lester, and Yarvis (2010).

Because the Air Force commissioned this research specifically to address individuals' capacity to be resilient and thus their well-being, our reports do not address whether or how fitness in each of the eight TFF domains could be linked to other outcomes of interest to the military. These include performance, military discipline, unit readiness, personnel costs, attrition, or retention. Those worthy topics were beyond this project's scope.

Some other important parameters shaped the literature reviews. First, across the study, we focused on research from the previous decade. Older studies were included, particularly landmark research that still defines the landscape or in which a particular line of inquiry has been dormant in recent years. Second, we prioritized research on adults in the United States. Research on children was included where germane (e.g., in discussions of family as a form of social support), and, occasionally, research on adults in other Western nations was referenced or subsumed within a large study. We generally excluded research on elderly populations. Third, we prioritized literature reviews, meta-analyses, and on-going bodies of research over more singular, smaller-scale studies.

The search for evidence on ways to promote resilience in each domain included actions that both individuals and organizations could take, such as information campaigns, policies, directives, programs, initiatives, facilities, or other resources. We did not filter out evidence related to Air Force practices under way, as the service was interested both in research on existing practices and studies that might suggest new paths to promote resilience. Our aim was not to collect examples of creative or promising initiatives at large but to seek scholarly publications assessing the stress-buffering capacity of initiatives. This collection of reviews, thus, generally does not address initiatives not yet evaluated for their effect.

The following sections bring together the TFF domain definitions and highlights of the resilience-related constructs and interventions described in the eight literature review reports cited above. The full reviews and complete bibliographies for each are provided in the eight peer-reviewed reports, and interested readers should examine those reports to gain more insights into, details about, and references for each individual TFF domain.

Medical Fitness[11]

Definition

Medical fitness is being medically capable "to perform duties under all conditions without excessive loss of quality of life, excessive loss of duty time or separation from duty, aggravation of existing medical conditions, or endangering the health of others" (Shih, Meadows, and Martin, 2013, p. 5). This means that service members are free from medical conditions or vulnerabilities that would limit their readiness.

---

[11] Excerpted from Shih, Meadows, and Martin (2013).

Key Resilience Constructs and Factors

Key resilience factors within the medical domain can be grouped into four categories:

- *preventive care* (e.g., routine physical exams, immunizations, screening for hearing, vision, and dental problems)
- *facilitators and barriers to accessing appropriate, quality health care* (e.g., health insurance, affordability of health care, health care provider staffing, stigma, geography)
- *the presence and management of injuries and wounds* (e.g., traumatic injury, traumatic brain injury, chronic pain)
- *the presence and management of chronic conditions* (e.g., obesity, diabetes, respiratory problems).

Gold standards exist for some measures of medical fitness, especially as they pertain to certain chronic diseases. But for other conditions, such as perceptions of pain, measures are more subjective. Measures of self-rated health are popular. The data are easy to collect and have been linked to depressive symptoms, health-related quality of life, risk of adverse clinical outcomes, and mortality. Research has shown that the key constructs within medical fitness can buffer stress; lack of these can make it harder to cope with stress.

Interventions to Promote Medical Fitness

Interventions that promote regular preventive care and encourage positive health behaviors, or that curb negative ones, may be particularly effective at staving off medical conditions that can compromise resiliency and military (medical) readiness. These interventions may be most feasible to administer through telephone, mobile text messaging, the Internet, and worksite health and wellness programs (HWPs). Industry standard programs include health risk assessments, health coaching, education classes, web resources, employee assistance programs, and fitness centers. HWPs have been linked to increased employee health by reducing dietary fat intake, high blood pressure, high cholesterol, and tobacco use. Such programs provide employers a return on investment through reductions in health care costs (e.g., insurance claims) and reduced absenteeism and increased worker productivity. Behavior change interventions, frequently used in HWPs, are increasingly using electronic media (e.g., email, Internet, Short Message Service [SMS], or text messages) to convey information or reminders to participants.

Nutritional Fitness[12]

Definition

Nutritional fitness can be defined as consuming "the nutrients needed to facilitate not only good health and readiness but also resilience against the physical and mental stressors associated with military service" (Flórez, Shih, and Martin, 2014, p. 5).

Key Resilience Constructs and Factors

Key resilience factors include the following:

- *Individual food intake* includes the frequency of consumption, portion size, dietary supplements, fat intake, and restaurant eating; real-time measures or estimates of past consumption can be translated into nutrient constituents of the food (e.g., amount of certain vitamins, calories, and fat).
- *Food choice motivations, barriers, and knowledge* refer not only food intake but also to food self-efficacy (e.g., how much a person is able to adopt attitudes and behaviors that could improve his/her health status related to nutrition), self-rated preferences, convenience, price, mood difficulties with modifying eating habits, and general nutritional knowledge.
- *Food environment* encompasses the nutrition, availability, quality, and cost of specific foods accessible in homes, schools, restaurants, vending machines, and grocery stores.
- *Biomarkers* of nutritional fitness indicate the presence (or absence) of specific nutrients in the body; these biomarkers can be used to estimate diet-disease risk factors.

The Western diet is characterized by consumption of excess calories and the prevalence of processed and fried foods, sugar, refined grains, high-fat animal-based protein, and alcohol. Eating is often an impulsive, automatic behavior that can be stimulated by food cues (e.g., plate size, cookies by the cash register). Further, the association between diet and stress is often reciprocal: Diet can affect the body's ability to deal with stress, and stress can influence diet.

There is a growing body of research on the role of nutrition in brain functioning and mental and physical health. For example, low vitamin D levels have been linked to cognitive impairment, depression, bipolar disorder, schizophrenia, softening of the bones, and increased risk of injury among athletes. Obese children are more prone to develop mood disorders (e.g., depression and anxiety), are less likely to be able to curb impulsive behavior, and report more symptoms of social withdrawal and isolation.

Interventions to Promote Nutritional Fitness

Interventions aimed at improving dietary fitness occur at three levels: individual, environment, and community. Individual-level interventions focus on individual eating

---

[12] Excerpted from Flórez, Shih, and Martin (2014).

behaviors, typically through some type of behavioral counseling, which can range from a single session to more than 20 sessions over a two-year period. Environment-level interventions focus on increasing access to healthful foods, modifying consumption cues in one's environment (e.g., smaller plates), and introducing dietary-related communication campaigns. Community or context-specific interventions can be provided in settings where people spend most of their time (work, school, and faith-based organizations). Examples include reducing portion sizes in cafeterias, raising prices in vending machines, and showing nutritional videos. Interventions at all levels can use nutritional education as a component of the program (e.g., providing evidence supporting or rejecting diet and supplement claims, teaching the long-term health consequences of poor nutritional choices).

Environmental Fitness[13]

Definition

Environmental fitness can be defined as the knowledge, skills, and behaviors necessary to successfully protect oneself from stress associated with one's environment or to successfully withstand the stressors that are encountered.

Key Resilience Constructs and Factors

Examples of environmental stressors include physical stressors (e.g., temperature, noise, altitude) and chemical stressors (e.g., occupational and environmental contaminants, including exposure to jet propellant fuel).[14] Key resilience factors in this TFF domain are grouped into two categories:

- *Prevention* addresses those aspects to mitigate environmental stress and hazards before they are encountered by personnel.
- *Protection* addresses mitigating environmental stress during the time the stress or hazards affect personnel.

Lack of environmental fitness can result in lack of resilience in the face of such stressors and lead to workplace-related injuries. In the military, the "workplace" would encompass not only military installations but also field exercises, domestic and overseas missions, and military transport to and from those destinations.

Traditional objective measures of occupational safety and health (e.g., deaths, injuries, and illness resulting from environmental stressors) have been enhanced by the development of measures of safety culture and climate, which can serve as early warning indicators of emerging

---

[13] Excerpted from Shih et al. (2015).

[14] Biological stressors, such as food, water, and vector-borne disease, are addressed in the medical fitness domain report (Shih, Meadows, and Martin, 2013).

problems. With prevention practices, a management commitment to safety has been demonstrated to be key to positive resilience-related outcomes. Safety training and education can have an effect if *targeted* at specific behaviors (e.g., using safety goggles) rather than at safety in general. No evidence links financial incentives to increased safety or reduced accidents or injuries. Safety inspections with corporate penalties reduce workplace injuries only in the short term, especially if they are associated with use of personal protective equipment (PPE); however, compliance with safety standards is not always linked to a reduction in workplace injury.

With protective practices, the effectiveness of PPE depends largely on whether it is used properly and if it is job- or industry-specific. Acclimatization and tolerance can reduce the negative effect of certain environmental stressors, such as temperature and altitude. Workplace ergonomics are associated with preventing musculoskeletal problems and reducing injuries, workers' compensation claims, and lost workdays.

Interventions to Promote Environmental Fitness

Appropriate use of PPE is the most directly relevant environment fitness factor in preventing workplace injury. A number of factors influence compliance with PPE standards, including individual-level factors (e.g., sociodemographic characteristics, attitudes and beliefs, knowledge, and education), job-level factors (e.g., experience level, skill, cognitive demands, workload, work stress), and organizational-level factors (e.g., training, peer review, management support, safety, and culture climate).

Physical Fitness[15]

Definition

In the context of TFF, our study defined physical fitness "as a set of health or performance-related attributes relating to the activities and condition of the body" (Robson, 2013, p. 5).

Key Resilience Constructs and Factors

Key resilience factors include work- and health-related activities:

- *physical activities* and their associated mechanical (movement) or metabolic (aerobic or anaerobic) properties
- *physical abilities* such as strength, endurance, and quality of movement.

Physical fitness constructs can relate either to ability to perform demanding physical tasks (performance-related fitness) or promotion of general health and well-being (health-related fitness). Science is moving away from fitness standards based on population norms (e.g.,

---

[15] Excerpted from Robson (2013).

percentiles) to standards based on health-related outcomes, such as reduced morbidity, onset of chronic conditions (e.g., high blood pressure, diabetes), and mortality.

Self-reported measures of physical activity can be captured through activity diaries, logs, and surveys; these typically are unreliable and inaccurate. Objective methods include direct observation and use of devices such as pedometers, accelerometers/electronic motion sensors, and heart rate monitors. Many physical fitness tests have been developed to represent various physical ability constructs, including the one-mile walk, 1.5-mile run, the half sit-up test, pushups, pullups, the bench press, leg extensions, and bicep curls.

Physical activity can provide considerable benefits to both physical and mental health and can buffer stress's negative effects. Physical activity is strongly linked to medical fitness, physical fitness, and behavioral fitness (e.g., better sleep), and it can protect against depression and anxiety and increase self-esteem. Those less fit may see even greater benefits from physical activity than those who are more fit.

Interventions to Promote Physical Fitness

Interventions to promote physical fitness are clustered in three areas. *Informational approaches* are designed to motivate, promote, and maintain behavior primarily by targeting cognition and knowledge about physical activity and its benefits. *Behavioral and social approaches* foster the development of behavioral management skills and modifying the social environment to support changes in behavior. *Environmental and policy approaches* aim to increase opportunities to be physically active within communities.

Social Fitness[16]

Definition

Social fitness is the ability of service members to develop and maintain social relationships that they can draw on to manage stressors and to perform their duties successfully (Cacioppo, Reis, and Zautra, 2011). "Social fitness *resources* are the aspects of those relationships that strengthen a person's ability to withstand and rebound from challenges (e.g., stress, threat, or disaster) or even grow from them" (McGene, 2013, p. vii).

Key Resilience Constructs and Factors

The key resilience factor associated with social fitness is social support derived from family, friends, co-workers (including military units), physical communities and neighborhoods, cyber communities, and social groups with which a person identifies and to which he or she feels a sense of belonging. Social support can be characterized as occurring in three forms:

---

[16] Excerpted from McGene (2013).

- *emotional*, such as having someone to talk to about problems
- *instrumental*, such as a getting a loan or a ride to a doctor's appointment
- *informational*, for example, shared knowledge about which companies are hiring.

Support can be actual or perceived. There is some evidence that perceived support is more influential for mental health than actual received support. Facilitators of social support include cohesion, group stability, and positive interactions and communication. In contrast, inhibitors of social support include group discord and conflict, geographic mobility, and bullying and ostracism. Family support has been demonstrated to be particularly important for resilience and psychological well-being.

Measures of individual-level social support are typically survey scales. At the neighborhood or community level, available social support is widely measured not only through survey data but also through indicators of lack of social ties and resources, such as crime, poverty, and high residential turnover.

Interventions to Improve Social Fitness

Social support can be promoted by various means. Economically disadvantaged individuals could benefit from access to networks promoting in-kind assistance among neighborhood or community members (e.g., exchanging babysitting for home repairs). Perceptions of social support actually may be cognitive distortions (e.g., no one cares or no one would help me) that could be addressed through psychological counseling. Interventions that promote social skills and more frequent and constructive social interactions (e.g., communication, mutual exchange) and that reduce conflict and group division (e.g., integration) can help develop social fitness, too. Geographic mobility is a potential barrier to social support in military populations, and interventions that use cyber or virtual communities (e.g., social media, video chat) may be especially useful tools to increase social connection and social support.

Spiritual Fitness[17]

Definition

Spiritual fitness can be defined as "the capacity for adherence to core personal values (i.e., a belief system) that reflect beliefs in transcendent or ultimate meaning and purpose" (Yeung and Martin, 2013, p. 6). It is important to note that "spiritual fitness does not require any degree of religiosity or belief in the supernatural. Atheists who hold a secular philosophy of meaning and purpose can be spiritually fit as well" (Yeung and Martin, 2013, p. 5).

---

[17] Excerpted from Yeung and Martin (2013).

Key Resilience Constructs and Factors

Self-administered survey scales and clinician assessment tools provide measures of constructs of spirituality, which have shown links to individual resilience and well-being. Key resilience factors fall into four categories:

- a *spiritual worldview* that includes beliefs in life's purpose and meaning, transcendence, and personal values
- *personal religious or spiritual practices and rituals* (e.g., prayer, meditation)
- *social support from a spiritual or religious community*
- *spiritual or religious coping* in which individuals use their beliefs as a source of comfort to deal with stress and strain.

Spiritual fitness has been linked to well-being in multiple ways. First, possessing a sense of meaning and purpose in life is strongly and positively associated with psychological well-being and perceived quality of life. It can offer a way for people to cope with trauma. Second, personal religious and spiritual rituals and practices are linked to improved physical and mental health (e.g., lower anxiety and depression, fewer physical indicators of stress, decreased substance use). Spiritual meditation also may improve health, buffering physiological stress and increasing pain tolerance. Third, there is converging, albeit indirect, evidence that individuals who have support from a spiritual community experience benefits to their health and well-being. Finally, use of spiritual beliefs to cope with stressors can drive PTG and improve mental health. Religious coping that is positive (e.g., focused on forgiveness) is associated with better mental health outcomes, and negative religious coping (e.g., focused on punishment from God or the devil's role) is associated with worse outcomes. Spiritual coping appears to be less effective in coping with such physical stressors as pain. Most of the empirical evidence indicates that several constructs of spiritual fitness can protect against suicide.

Interventions to Improve Spiritual Fitness

Many of the spiritual interventions evaluated by research are programs focused on instilling a sense of meaning and purpose in life. Diverse types of spiritual interventions, including training, counseling, prayer, mindfulness, meditation, spiritual leadership, and spiritual caregiving, have been linked to improved resilience and well-being. The importance of cultural appropriateness of the interventions is also emphasized in this literature.

Behavioral Fitness[18]

Definition

This study defined behavioral fitness as "conduct, routines, and habits that promote health and well-being." Because almost any health "behavior" could be included in this domain, we included those addressed in the behavioral fitness article in the special TFF issue of *Military Medicine* (Bray et al., 2010). We restricted it to only those behaviors that did not fall under any of the other seven TFF domains.

Key Resilience Constructs and Factors

Key resilience factors include the following:

- *Sleep behaviors* are critical to physical and psychological functioning. Excessive sleep loss can contribute to chronic health conditions, poor mental health, and reduced adaptability to stress.
- *Alcohol and drug use disorders* can negatively affect physical and mental health. Heavy drinking has been linked strongly to various negative health outcomes, including stroke, depression, sleep disorders, heart disease, cancer, and immune system deficiency. Moderate drinking has some health benefits, especially for cardiovascular health. Alcohol use can have stress-buffering effect, but regular intoxication may lead to addiction. Numerous studies have found that both acute and chronic stresses are associated with risk of drug addiction.
- *Smoking* can cause many chronic health conditions, including cancer, respiratory disease, cardiovascular disease, gastrointestinal disease, and reproductive problems. Less well known, smoking also can increase stress and the risk for mood and panic disorders. Smoking cessation can increase stress in the short term but overall is associated with decreased stress and reduced risk of these disorders. However, stress levels may contribute to maintenance and relapse of smoking behavior.

Sleep measures include self-reports on questionnaires, wrist-worn actigraph devices to detect motion, and invasive physiological tests conducted in a sleep lab. Research relies largely on self-reported measures of alcohol and drug use, although toxicology screens may be employed as well. Self-reports of smoking are common, but a more accurate measure is a biomarker found in such bodily fluids as saliva.

Interventions to Improve Behavioral Fitness

Sleep issues can be effectively addressed with good sleep hygiene behaviors, behavioral therapies, and medication when necessary. Research has found that behavioral therapies, sometimes combined with medications, can be effective in treating addiction to drugs or alcohol.

---

[18] Excerpted from Robson and Salcedo (2014).

Price increases have been shown to be one of the most effective strategies for the prevention of smoking and alcohol consumption.

Many factors are associated with successful changes in health behaviors such as these, including motivation, attitudes, family background, knowledge, health insurance, and social networks. Interventions to promote health behavior should be individually tailored and target high-risk individuals using multimodal means of communication (e.g., in-person, text messages, emails). Realistic expectations about the ability to change health-related behavior are essential.

Psychological Fitness[19]

Definition

Psychological fitness is defined as the integration and optimization of cognitive processes and abilities, behaviors, and emotions to positively affect performance, well-being, and response to stress.[20]

Key Resilience Constructs and Factors

The psychological literature on resilience is extensive and long-standing. Key resilience factors fall into three categories:[21]

- *Cognitive factors* include measures reflecting individuals' thoughts and beliefs about themselves (e.g., self-efficacy, self-esteem) in addition to interpretations of their situation (e.g., perceived control).
- *Affective factors* include the experience of positive and negative emotions (e.g., positive and negative affect, optimism).
- *Self-regulation factors* include measures of self-regulation and control (e.g., coping strategies).

Measurement of psychological constructs is primarily done by self-report survey or questionnaire; self-regulation most often has been measured in laboratory settings. Research has found that self-efficacy is associated with whether one experiences a challenge as stressful and that perception of lack of efficacy can itself induce stress. Individuals who believe that they have

---

[19] Excerpted from Robson (2014).

[20] This is a slightly modified version of the definition that appeared in the psychological fitness domain article in the special TFF issue of *Military Medicine* (Bates et al., 2010).

[21] Mental health is included in this domain. As noted in the psychological fitness report: "Although background (e.g., childhood trauma, socioeconomic status) and psychological disorders including depression, anxiety, and post-traumatic stress disorder (PTSD) can be a sign of poor psychological resilience and may also make people more vulnerable to stress, these topics are not the primary focus of this report. Extensive research has been conducted on these topics with dedicated attention to understanding these problems in military populations and evidence-based interventions.... Therefore, the focus of this report is on the psychological resources that can promote resilience" (Robson, 2014, p. 6).

little control over events and their own behavior are at higher risk for depression and anxiety, respond poorly to stress, and demonstrate less happiness than those who perceive an internal locus of control. Positive affect is associated with a host of benefits (e.g., confidence, optimism, pro-social behavior, immunity, and physical well-being) that can help individuals be resilient in the face of adversity. Self-regulation facilitates the ability to exercise restraint, direct choices, and persist in the face of adversity. It also is important in helping individuals to bounce back after experiencing stress. Research has shown that different coping strategies can have different outcomes for well-being. No coping strategy is beneficial for all individuals in all situations. It is also important to note that all of these psychological resilience factors can be affected by a number of other factors, including experiences with prior and recent stress, social support, and health behaviors (e.g., smoking, drinking).

Interventions to Improve Psychological Fitness

Common themes across interventions to promote psychological fitness include two components. The first factor is *self-awareness*, which involves the identification of how individuals respond to stress, emotions they experience, and their thought processes. The second factor is *skill building*—the promotion of positive emotions, happiness, confidence, self-esteem, and well-being.

Given that much of the research on psychological resilience conducted to date is correlational and correlation does not imply causation, it is important to keep in mind that interventions to promote psychological fitness may not be as effective as anticipated if they do not also address other factors. Pessimistic thinking may decrease happiness; however, another factor (e.g., job loss) actually may be responsible for both. Thus, the best approach to building psychological resources may require specificity in both the needs of a defined population as well as the type of stressors that they commonly experience.

Conclusion

Scientific research has identified constructs across the eight TFF domains that are associated with stress, including the

- risk of experiencing stress
- interpretation of an event as stressful
- physiological reaction to an event as stressful
- ability to manage or cope with stress
- the ability to bounce back or even grow from a stressful experience.

Not all disciplines or scholars use the word "resilience" when studying stress, so a review of the relevant research must not be bound to that word as a search term. These eight domains were selected by DoD as a way to conceptualize a diverse approach to resilience that focuses on both the body and the mind. There is no body of scholarship that has empirically determined that these are the "correct" eight domains. Other scholars or institutions may organize their approaches to holistic well-being differently. These domains can be matched to the Air Force's four pillars of well-being: mental, physical, social, and spiritual. None are mutually exclusive, and at times our study had to make a judgment call about which reports should cover which overlapping topics.

The literature reviews examined research in each domain on constructs, measures, and direct and buffering links to stress and physical and mental well-being. Key resilience-related constructs across the fitness domains are often measured through self-reports, whether through individuals' filling out questionnaires or clinician-administered assessments. This is particularly true for large-scale studies. Many of these scales or screenings have already undergone significant development and testing. Typically much more costly and time-consuming are objective measures of individual fitness and stress-response assessed through devices or biological tests or screenings (e.g., sleep studies, blood tests, urinalysis). Community- and neighborhood-level assessments may include collective indicators of fitness or lack of fitness (e.g., accident rates, high residential turnover, accessibility, affordability of high-quality food).

Often, the interventions that have been shown to be effective in promoting fitness in the eight TFF domains target specific behaviors or the specific needs of individuals rather than broadly addressing an entire population or an entire range of behaviors. Information and communication technologies can be used to convey reminders for check-ups and screenings, send messages to support behavioral changes, and sustain social networks after geographic relocation. Some interventions are designed to interact directly with individuals, such as health coaching and individual psychological or spiritual counseling. Other interventions are focused on creating an environment that provides many opportunities for fitness-promoting behaviors and reduces temptation to make unhealthy choices (e.g., providing exercise and recreational facilities; designing ergonomic work stations; sponsoring social activities to help build and maintain social networks; setting higher prices for alcohol, tobacco, and junk food, reducing plate sizes in restaurants and cafeterias).

4. Resilience-Related Air Force Data

These reviews of the scientific literature on resilience and the TFF domains seek to support Air Force efforts to understand and define resilience and to determine how to measure and track it. To develop recommendations relevant for the Air Force, we needed to understand not only what has been documented in the scientific literature but also which Air Force information and programs were already in existence.

In 2010, when the Air Force Resilience Office (now Comprehensive Airman Fitness Office) was established in the office of Air Force Services, the staff looked to develop metrics to track the resilience of the force. We proposed drawing on previously validated scales to develop an instrument that could assess the force along the eight domains of TFF. But Air Force leaders at that time were working to reduce the survey burden on the Air Force population. Instead, the research sponsors requested that we characterize the degree to which existing measures could help them assess resilience.

We investigated whether we could evaluate the actual, existing data on Air Force personnel and their families against what the literature suggests are suitable indicators of resiliency. Sources would have included Air Force medical, personnel, and survey data. This effort could have resulted in revisions to the types of data the Air Force collects or recommendations for more data collection and sharing. Ultimately, this endeavor proved infeasible because of the many requirements involved in accessing such a diverse array of data, including sensitive information protected by the Privacy Act of 1974 and the Health Insurance Portability and Accountability Act (HIPAA). The data also were "owned" by many different organizations, further complicating our ability to synthesize them.

Barriers existed not just for us but to information-sharing across the different organizations that hold data of potential relevance for tracking resilience resources. HIPAA regulations govern disclosure of protected health information, the Privacy Act of 1974 governs dissemination of personally identifiable information in personnel records, and human subjects research protection protocols may limit the sharing of data collected for research purposes. Data exchanges also take additional resources both to package and send data, as well as to understand and interpret data received from other offices. Finally, there were cultural norms about data ownership that restricted sharing to only the office requesting the data collection (e.g., the office that sponsored a survey).

For the purposes of this study, we learned more about the different measures even where we had access only to internal aggregate data reports, survey instruments, or record descriptions. Overall, we found that the greatest amount of data was available for the active component. Less information was collected about guard and reserve Airmen; the least information was available for family members and Air Force civilians. We also caution the reader that no single data source is perfectly suited for the purposes of tracking resilience or TFF among Airmen, their families, and civilian Airmen. We have organized the resilience-related data according to type and source:

- behavioral incidents that come to the attention of the Air Force that may serve as signs of lack of resilience
- evaluations or assessments by professionals in the Air Force
- self-reports of Airmen who volunteer in Air Force or DoD surveys capturing a range of resilience-related information
- Air Force personnel and incident data that indicate potential stressors.

Behavioral Incidents

Across the military, commonly tracked behavioral incidents are data sources that focus on the negative, or indicators of the absence of resilience factors. These metrics include the following:

- driving under the influence (DUI) statistics
- suicide rates and suicide event report statistics
- domestic violence reports
- positive drug tests
- accidents
- criminal behavior.

Such statistics could be indicators of poor self-regulation, negative emotions, maladaptive or lack of coping strategies, poor safety culture or climate, and other resilience factors. The intent of promoting resilience, of course, is to prevent Airmen, Air Force civilians, and Air Force family members from ever showing up in these statistics.

Statistics on the use of facilities, programs, and services are problematic as indicators of resilience, for several reasons. First, those accessing mental health services could be said to be lacking resilience because they needed professional help. But they also could be characterized as resilient, because they are drawing on mental health professionals to help them cope, in contrast, say, to those who might, instead, turn to drugs or alcohol. Second, these indicators of negative behavior alone also cannot tell us whether the behavior resulted from the individual's inability to cope with a stressful event. For example, use of recreational drugs may not be an indicator of ineffective coping for everyone.

Air Force Professional Assessments

Assessments by Air Force professionals also contain information related to the resilience constructs in TFF domains and the Air Force's pillars of well-being. Professional assessments of the broader population include administration of the physical fitness test, medical and dental examinations, and workplace safety inspections.

Target assessments of specific populations also exist. The Lackland Behavioral Questionnaire (LBQ) is a 61-item, multiple-choice, paper questionnaire administered to all Air Force military enlisted personnel within the first few days of basic military training (BMT). This assessment has been administered continuously since 2006, as a part of the Biographical Evaluation and Screening of Troops (BEST) program. The questionnaire responses are linked with individual identities: They are employed in combination with targeted follow-up interviews to identify trainees who might be in acute need of mental health care. The results are not shared with security clearance or sensitive occupation screenings or organizations that receive the recruits once they have completed BMT. In rare cases when a recruit refuses to fully participate in the latter phases of the BEST program, a minimum amount of LBQ information can be shared with BMT squadron commanders. Limited LBQ results also are entered into medical progress notes and are available to medical providers at the recruits' new units. The results have been assessed against subsequent behavioral, psychological, medical, and performance data.

The Pre-Deployment Health Assessment (pre-DHA) and Post Deployment Health Assessment/Reassessment (PDHA/PDHRA) ask Airmen questions before and after deployment to identify mental and behavioral health concerns. The assessment includes self-rated mental health, self-reported tobacco and alcohol use, symptoms of PTSD and depression, disruptive life stressors, exposure to combat or environmental threats (e.g., chemicals or smoke), wounds or injury during deployment, and generalized post-deployment physical symptoms. After Airmen complete the online form, a health care provider can assess the risk of harm to the Airman himself or to others; if necessary, the provider can help address problems or make referrals for further evaluation and treatment. Mental health evaluations are another type of professional assessment when a problem has been self-identified or identified in some other way and either requested or mandated.

Relevant Self-Report Air Force Survey Data

Many Air Force surveys contain information that provide insights into resilience resources, such as social support and health behaviors, stressors, and coping, as well as the degree to which the environment promotes TFF. Examples of these surveys and types of relevant items are the following:

- *Caring for People Survey* (formerly Quality of Life) includes items on facilities and services, sources of social support, income/finances, and life satisfaction. Participants include active and reserve component Airmen, Air Force civilian employees, retirees, and spouses.
- *Air Force Community Assessment Survey* includes questions on social support, social cohesion, community well-being, economic and financial stress, exercise frequency, self-rated health, depressive symptoms, the CD-RISC, and satisfaction. Participants include active and reserve component Airmen, Air Force civilian employees, and spouses.

- *Air Force Climate Survey* captures job satisfaction, trust in leadership, unit performance, recognition, and resources, which could be indicators of stress and potential social support within the unit. Participants include active and reserve component Airmen and Air Force civilian employees.
- *Support and Resiliency Inventory,* which includes extensive measures of social support (friends, family, units, neighbors, and religious organizations) and a resiliency profile comprising short scales on physical well-being, emotional well-being, personal safety, financial welfare, coping success, support for others, help-seeking orientation, ability to perform work duties, community participation, and satisfaction with military life. Participants include active and reserve component Airmen, Air Force civilian employees, and spouses.
- *Web Health Assessment (WebHA)* includes items related to overall health, medication use, dental health, chronic disease, exercise, nutrition, tobacco and alcohol use, family history, preventive services, reproductive health, injury prevention, mental health, eating disorder symptoms, anger management, self-rated spiritual or religious health, and life stressors. Participants include active and reserve component Airmen.

There also are innumerable unit, base, major command, and other Air Force surveys. Data on Air Force personnel are available in such DoD surveys as the Morale, Welfare and Recreation survey, the Defense Manpower Data Center Status of Forces Surveys, and the Active Duty Survey of Spouses. Response rates can vary by survey and subpopulations. Although many of the Air Force and DoD surveys are recurring, they are cross-sectional surveys. Longitudinal results for individuals, which might provide a good assessment of respondent self-reports pre- and post-stressors, are not tracked.

Air Force Personnel or Report Data That Indicate Potential Stressors

As noted earlier, resilience cannot be understood outside the context of stressors. Therefore, an overview of the resilience of the force should take into account potential stressors that challenge the population. Recall that positive events, such as promotions and marriages, can be stressors, too. Data in Air Force personnel administrative files include indicators of some possible sources of stress, such as

- relocation
- deployments (number, duration, and location)
- tours outside the continental United States (both accompanied and unaccompanied)
- the addition or subtraction of dependents (spouse, children)
- disciplinary action
- promotion
- command assignment.

Data on reported complaints and incidents of physical violence, harassment, discrimination, and abuse are also indicators of stressful experiences. These would include reports of sexual assault, equal opportunity complaints, and complaints filed with the inspector general. These data would need to be used in conjunction with another data source described in this chapter; knowledge of stressors or stressful situations experienced by an individual can help the Air Force to determine if, in fact, negative behavioral outcomes, professional assessments, or self-report data are the results of unsuccessful adaptation to stress and perhaps indicative of a lack of resilience in the force.

Assessing Air Force Resilience

In this chapter, we have shown that there are a great number of sources of data with relevance for understanding resilience resources in the Air Force. These data are complementary, as they cover different types of stressors, different resilience resource constructs within the eight TFF domains, different levels of assessment (e.g., individuals, communities), and multiple types of data (e.g., behavioral metrics, professional assessments, potential stressors, survey self-reports). But this information is spread across many diverse datasets owned by many different organizations. Data protections, legal and regulatory requirements (such as the Privacy Act and HIPAA), and the sheer labor required to merge all these data make it difficult if not impossible to accomplish such a task.

5. Promoting Resilience in the Air Force

The Air Force focus on resilience stems from leaders' concern about the effect of the wartime mission on psychological health, suicide rates, and families. Much of the Air Force's organic, long-standing institutional capability supports resilience. For example, the chaplain corps, medical centers, and recreational facilities all can support resilience.

Since the attacks of September 11, Air Force leaders increasingly have focused on supporting the psychological domain. The Air Force has strengthened counseling and medical approaches to psychological well-being. These efforts have concentrated on reducing stigma for mental health care and increasing access to mental health care providers. The Air Force also has expanded efforts to sustain performance and promote resilience before individuals and families are in distress. Examples of specific programs and initiatives relevant for resilience that were developed since the September 11 attacks include the following:

- *Airman Resilience Training* is an educational briefing designed to improve Airmen's psychological reactions to stress during and after deployment and to encourage the use of mental health services among those who could potentially benefit.
- The *Deployment Transition Center* is a facility for Airmen returning home from deployments where they were "regularly exposed to significant risk of death in direct combat or regularly exposed to traumatic events" (USAF, 2014, p. 5).
- The *Air Force Wounded Warrior Program* helps combat- or hostilities-related wounded, ill, or injured Airmen with the transition to either a successful return to duty or to the civilian community.
- *Wingman Day* is an annual (now biannual) Air Force–wide, unit-level event with activities that "emphasize informational awareness, accountability, team-building, and communication skills for selected topics" (USAF, 2014), which may include suicide prevention, safety, resilience, and health and well-being.
- *Military Family Life Consultants,* a DoD initiative, are nonmilitary licensed counselors assigned to Air Force installations for 180-day terms to provide free, nonmedical, short-term, situational problem-solving counseling to Airmen and their families. This program expanded the resources available to service members by offering an alternative to military mental health care providers.
- *Master Resilience Trainers* provide training in skills that support the Air Force's four domains of fitness.

When developing recommendations to help the Air Force promote resilience, we considered the particular Air Force context and Air Force Resilience Office priorities and the resources that already existed that could be leveraged (to avoid unnecessary cost or duplication). We also took into account what we learned from literature reviews in the eight domains of TFF.

RAND Project AIR FORCE Recommendations

In Chapter 3, we included examples of lessons that can be drawn from the eight TFF literature reviews regarding domain-specific interventions. This research project also provided the following Air Force–specific recommendations in 2011 for it to consider while building its program to support resilience across the Air Force community. These recommendations were informed by discussions with the research sponsors, by previous research conducted for the Air Force, by opportunities to review types of internal Air Force data described in Chapter 4, and by U.S. population trends identified in the domain-specific literature reviews. Our recommendations are based on what appeared to be the greatest gaps or opportunities for improvement.

Promote Regular Unit Physical Activity

Physical activity has many direct and buffering benefits to the health, well-being, and readiness of the force, as noted in Chapter 3 and the companion report on physical fitness (Robson, 2013). Physical activity is strongly linked to better medical fitness (e.g., cardiorespiratory health, reduced risks for some cancers), physical fitness (e.g., body composition, muscular fitness), psychological fitness (e.g., stress-buffering, protection against depression and anxiety; increased self-esteem), and behavioral fitness (e.g., sleep hygiene, sleep quality) (see Figure 5.1). Group physical activity can also improve social fitness through the development of social networks and cohesion.

To help convey the importance of physical fitness and to institutionalize physical activity across the Air Force, we recommended holding commanders accountable for the physical fitness of their military personnel, which is measured twice a year. Existing methods for holding commanders accountable for the readiness, work performance, and behavior of their Airmen

Figure 5.1. Physical Activity Can Boost Fitness Across a Number of Domains

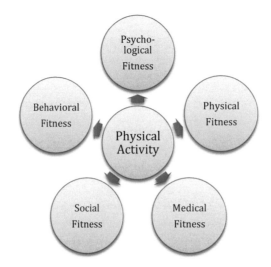

could be extended to include Airmen's physical fitness. In this manner, commanders can develop strategies for meeting fitness goals that match the needs of their personnel, and physical fitness can become integrated as a part of an Airman's duties, rather than be in competition with them.

We also recommended that the Air Force promote organized regular physical activity in work groups, which may include both Air Force military and civilian personnel. These institutional habits could provide stress relief, build unit cohesion, foster social support for a fit lifestyle, and promote physical and psychological well-being, particularly for those in sedentary jobs. We were not suggesting that all units must run, lift weights, or do exercises in unison. Leaders should think creatively about diverse activities with an aerobic component, such as walking, basketball, ultimate Frisbee, batting cages, tai chi, and obstacle race challenges. More rigorous activities may be appropriate, depending on the overall fitness of the unit. It is also important to remember that physical activity includes more than just aerobic activities. It can also include walking, yoga, bowling, dancing, and gardening, and these activities can be very beneficial for sedentary, injured or ill, obese, and exercise-averse populations. These also might be provided as social activities where family members would be welcome, too. This could promote physical activity among family members and strengthen family ties, reduce work-family conflict, and help maintain social support as a resilience resource.

Physical activity can help reduce the major risks to optimal mission performance: physical injury, being overweight, and psychosocial dysfunction. The contributions of physical fitness to resilience make it a smart investment, even in times of scarce resources.

Better Resource Health and Wellness Centers to Increase Capacity for Community and Targeted Interventions by Subject Matter Experts

Given the paramount importance of physical fitness for resilience and overall well-being (Robson, 2013), we also recommended a greater commitment of resources to Health and Wellness Centers (HAWCs). At the time of this study, there were 77 HAWCs in the Air Force. The authorized staff per base included one health educator, one registered dietician, an exercise physiologist, and an office manager. If the installation had more than 5,000 active duty personnel assigned, the HAWC also was authorized one health fitness technician/specialist. As noted in several of the literature reviews in this series (see Chapter 3), effective interventions to promote fitness and support healthy habits often need to be individualized or specific and not just general information campaigns. HAWCs were already designed to contain the expertise, medical oversight, and access to facilities essential to provide such services as

- health education
- health coaching
- personalized dietary and fitness plans
- group fitness challenges or events
- physical activity classes (e.g., yoga, kick boxing)
- health campaigns.

Thus, these centers can enhance individual readiness and fitness across multiple domains (physical, nutritional, behavioral, medical, social), which can in turn benefit psychological well-being. We cannot emphasize enough the role that physical health can play in psychological health.

Unfortunately, HAWCs often lack sufficient personnel and resources to successfully serve an installations' active duty populations. According to information provided by the Air Force, line-funded fill rates for each position ranged from 62 to 91 percent. In total, there were only 364 staff for approximately 330,000 active duty Airmen. We recommended fully staffing and resourcing the HAWCs at least to meet the needs of the active duty population, if not the total force and family members as well.

Continue to Leverage Wingman Day

Wingman Day initially was timed to precede the winter holidays when accidents and other negative outcomes tended to increase. Its common themes had included prevention of DUIs and motor vehicle accidents, suicide prevention, and Airmen getting to know and look out for one another (i.e., being a good "wingman"). Some units and installations organize health fairs as part of their events. We recommended that the Air Force headquarters look for opportunities and creative ways to promote the following, which are all resilience factors discussed in Chapter 3 and the eight companion TFF reports, among its suggested Wingman Day topics and activities:

- group physical activities
- good sleep hygiene
- instilling a safety culture and habit of PPE use
- conflict resolution skills
- social cohesion and sense of belonging in the Air Force and the work group
- stress management skills: self-awareness of one's responses to stress, healthy alternatives if needed or advisable
- healthy diets, to include dispelling myths and providing accurate information about the true benefits and health risks of the latest diet fads, energy drinks, and supplements.

We do not suggest that units have not already taken up these topics. A desirable feature of Wingman Day is that commanders can tailor topics to match local needs rather than be constrained by standardized activities mandated by Air Force headquarters. Local planning and preparation have received headquarters support in suggested themes and prepared ideas and materials—it was toward that end that we recommended ways to incorporate constructs from across TFF domains.

Add a Programs and Services Tab to the Air Force Base Website Template

Some standardization of Air Force base websites is achieved through a website template. At the time of this study, during our review of Air Force programs targeting resilience (see Chapter 2), the research team found it difficult to locate information on base websites about local programs and services that can help Airmen and their families cope with stressors and build their resilience resources (e.g., the chaplain, mental health care providers, the sexual assault response coordinator, HAWCs). When our team sought local program information, the website search function often returned merely a local news story on a program or service (such as a story on a staffer receiving an award) and not contact and other essential information for which an Air Force community member might be searching. The lack of prominence and easy access to such information could present hurdles for new Air Force personnel, new spouses, those who just relocated to an installation, and leaders who need to access or recommend program support to assist unit or family members.

We recommended that the Air Force add a Programs and Services tab to the menu at the top of the installation website template. There could be other ways to accomplish the primary goal of establishing a standard location on each website so that Airmen and their family members can locate essential information (e.g., a link at the top right corner of every web page). This includes what each program or service offers, eligibility, level of confidentiality afforded, hours available, phone numbers (including DSN and commercial), address, and email link.

Increase the Sharing of Resilience-Related Data Across the Air Staff

Because there is currently untapped potential for measuring Air Force–wide resilience in existing Air Force data sources (see Chapter 4), RAND recommended that the Air Force promote information-sharing across Air Staff organizations whose functions address aspects of Air Force resiliency. These organizations are members of the Community Action Information Board (CAIB), which is designed to facilitate information-sharing and collective problem-solving. Some metrics are already tracked by the CAIB (e.g., suicide rates). But others were not necessarily shared (such as some survey results and aggregate statistics on professional assessments). Sharing helps to ensure that programming meets population needs and reduces duplication in data collection efforts. If feasible, given available resources and limitations on sharing individual-level data, we recommended that highly skilled Air Force analysts synthesize recent data from all sources to create resilience factor profiles, aggregated separately for active duty, guard, reserve, civilian, and spouse subpopulations.

Fill Gaps in Data Collection

The Air Force needs to understand pre- and poststress resilience factors to better target messaging and programs. The data collection efforts we reviewed in Chapter 4 were strong in certain areas (e.g., extensive information on tobacco use, symptoms of psychological distress) but they were lacking in others, based on resilience-related constructs and measures identified in the literature reviews. To fill gaps in Air Force–wide surveys' coverage of TFF domains, the Air Force could draw on measures already developed by researchers. After reviewing the empirical literature and examining the types of resilience-related data collected by the Air Force, we recommended expanding assessments of

- nutritional habits
- physical activity
- sleep hygiene
- the use of PPE
- the spiritual needs of secular members.

We refer readers to the nutritional, physical, behavioral, environmental, and spiritual fitness companion reports for further details about existing measures (Flórez, Shih, and Martin, 2014; Robson, 2013; Robson and Salcedo, 2014; Shih et al., 2015; Yeung and Martin, 2013).

Strengthen the Air Force Resilience Office's Ability to Promote Resilience Factors Across the Force

The Air Force Resilience Office (now Comprehensive Airman Fitness Office) was still in development at the time of this study, and it faced a challenge in deciding how to assess and promote resilience because it lacked sufficient, substantive expertise. We recommended that staff assignments to this office include a professional in each of the Air Force's physical, psychological, spiritual, and social domains so that all of the TFF domains have adequate representation. As we noted in Chapter 2, the eight domains of TFF (medical, nutritional, environmental, physical, social, spiritual, behavioral, and psychological) collectively influence an individual's ability to cope with stress, or their resiliency. These professionals need not all be military personnel, particularly if there are civilian employees who hold sufficient knowledge of Air Force personnel, organization, and culture that they can contextualize their efforts appropriately.

Because the office intended to evaluate the effect of resilience initiatives, we recommended the addition of a Ph.D.-level analyst with at least 10 years of experience and expertise in research design and program evaluation. This would enable the office to assess data strengths and weaknesses to appropriately qualify any results and to guide and support efforts to demonstrate the effectiveness of different programs and interventions. Although ideas intuitively may seem as if they would contribute to a desired outcome, it is important to identify efforts that consume resources and produce no perceptible positive results. Particularly in an era of increasing budget constraints, it is important that the Air Force be able to extract the most good from its investments.

Conclusion

For more than a decade, the Air Force has been strengthening and expanding its efforts to support the psychological well-being of Airmen and their family members. However, significant gains in the psychological realm could be made by expanding and institutionalizing efforts to promote physical health, too. RAND developed recommendations for the Air Force to enhance its ability to advance the resilience of the Air Force community and to develop a new Air Force office responsible for assessing and improving Air Force resilience.

This report concludes the RAND Project AIR FORCE series of reports on resiliency. It reviews the concept of resilience and resilience factors, and, in an appendix provides an extensive list of measures of resilience and the related concepts of hardiness and flourishing. This report provides highlights from the eight companion reports in this series, and from peer-reviewed literature reviews in each of the eight TFF domains, designed to be succinct and accessible to the nonspecialist. These other reports include examples of scientific measures of constructs and resilience factors in each domain. We also categorize the types of data the Air Force already was collecting at the time of this study that hold relevance for understanding the resilience of the force. Finally, we document the overarching recommendations we provided to the Air Force to help strengthen the new office responsible for resilience and to promote Airman and family resilience. To close, we would like to emphasize one important message.

There is no survey instrument, professional assessment, or biological test available today that would allow commanders to determine who in their unit will or will not be resilient in the face of stress. Predicting human behavior is extremely difficult. In social science, the best predictors tend to capture only a small percentage of the variance. Resilience is in a constant state of fluctuation; resilience resources and stressors can come and go. Individuals may be resilient in the face of some stressors, such as extreme temperatures, a divorce, or a command assignment. They may fail to be resilient under other circumstances, such as if their child dies or they lose a limb as the result of an improvised explosive device. Further, acceptable responses to stress are to some degree socially constructed and culturally and contextually specific: There is no objective standard, for example, for how long an individual might grieve a loss before being classified as lacking resilience.

What the literature does help us understand is how the Air Force can build individual and community capacity to be resilient by understanding which factors shape the experience and interpretation of stressors, responses to stressors, and associated changes to well-being and resilience resources, if any, following the event.

Appendix. Measures of Resilience, Hardiness, and Flourishing Among Adults, Children, and Adolescents

This appendix, drawn from the literature, provides an extensive list of measures of resilience and the related concepts of hardiness and flourishing. It also includes notes about their focus, reliability, validity, and source. Table A.1 examines measures of resilience and hardiness among adults, and Table A.2 looks at measures of flourishing among adults. Table A.3 provides information on measures of resilience and hardiness among children and adolescents, and Table A.4 describes measures of flourishing among children and adolescents.

Table A.1. Measures of Resilience and Hardiness Among Adults

Name of Measure	Description	Reliability	Validity	Notes	Citation
Response to Stressful Experiences Scale (RSES)	The RSES is a 22-item scale designed to measure individual differences in cognitive, emotional, and behavioral responses to stressful life events. The scale contains five factors: meaning-making and restoration, active coping, cognitive flexibility, spirituality, and self-efficacy.	Internal consistency for the overall scale was .92. Test-retest reliability was .87. Factor analysis confirmed the five factors, although the authors note that the factors do not represent stand-alone subscales.	Scores on the RSES were moderately, positively correlated with the CD-RISC. Higher scores on the RSES were associated with higher scores on unit and general social support scales and negatively associated with psychological distress and overall mental health.	New scale that has not seen frequent use in the literature. Sample used in scale validation study included a Marine Expeditionary Unit, an Army national Guard Infantry Division, and an Army National Guard combat aviation brigade with recent combat experience.	Johnson et al. (2011).
Trauma Resilience Scale (TRS)	The TRS is specifically designed to measure individual perceptions of protective factors that help people following exposure to violent events. Two versions of the TRS are available: a 48-item, four-factor version (problem-solving, relationships, optimism, and spirituality) and a 37-item, three-factor version (problem-solving, relationships, and optimism).	Internal consistency for the overall scale was .93, regardless of the number of factors.	The four-factor TRS was best supported by the data. Each subscale was correlated with existing measures of coping strategies, social relationships, optimism, and spirituality.	Has not seen frequent use in the literature.	Madsen and Abell (2010).

Name of Measure	Description	Reliability	Validity	Notes	Citation
Brief Resiliency Scale (BRS)	The six-item BRS is designed to measure an individual's ability to bounce back, or recover, from stress.	Internal consistency ranged from .69 to .91, depending on the subsample.[22] Test-retest reliability ranged from .62 to .69, depending on the subsample. Factor analysis yielded only one factor.	The BRS was a reliable measure of a unitary dimension of resilience defined as bouncing back or coping with stress. It was negatively associated with anxiety, depression, negative affect, and physical symptoms, controlling for other resilience measures, optimism, social support and Type D personality (high negative affect and high social inhibition).	Has not seen frequent use in the literature.	Smith et al. (2008).
Military Hardiness Scale (MHS)	The 18-item MHS reflects three components of military hardiness: military-specific commitment (i.e., a strong identity with the military and commitment to a mission), military-specific control (i.e., job control and personal influence on mission outcomes), and military-specific challenges (i.e., degree to which the individual exerts personal resources in response to operational demand).	Internal consistency for the overall scale was .90.	Among a sample of soldiers stationed in Germany and deployed to Kosovo on a peacekeeping mission, military hardiness was positively associated with psychological health but not physical health, both during deployment and 1–2 months after deployment. Soldiers with higher MHS scores reported lower levels of depressive symptoms. And in the face of stress, having a higher level of military hardiness was associated with a lower level of depressive symptoms.		Dolan and Adler (2006).

___

[22] The study used four subsamples to validate the BRS: two samples of undergraduate students, one sample of cardiac rehabilitation patients, and a clinical sample of women with and without fibromyalgia.

Name of Measure	Description	Reliability	Validity	Notes	Citation
Deployment Risk and Resilience Inventory (DRRI)	The DRRI assesses key psychosocial risk and resilience factors for military personnel and veterans deployed to war zones or other hazardous environments. It has 14 subscales: two predeployment factors, 10 deployment or war-zone factors, and two postdeployment factors. Four subscales—childhood and family environment, preparedness, and deployment and postdeployment social support—can be construed as measures of resilience. DRRI is intended to identify deployment-related factors that put veterans at risk for postdeployment problems or that serve as protective factors.	Internal consistency ranged from .67 to .91 among a telephone sample of veterans and .75 to .94 among a mail survey of veterans.	Among a sample of Gulf War veterans, risk and resilience factors in the DRRI were more strongly associated with psychological health than physical health or neurocognitive deficits. General harassment showed the strongest associations with PTSD, depression, and anxiety. Perceived threat and nuclear, biological, or chemical agent exposures had robust associations with all outcomes, relative to other subscales.	A number of studies have used the DRRI and that number is increasing.[23]	King et al. (2006).
Personal Views Survey III-R (PVS-III-R)	The PVS-III-R is designed to measure three constructs: commitment, control, and challenge.	Internal consistency varied by subscale: .69 for commitment, .57 for control, .73 for challenge. Additional samples of college students and professional business consultants yielded overall internal consistencies of .70 to .77. Factor analysis confirmed 3 subscales.	The PVS-III-R was negatively associated with repressive coping (e.g., denial or avoidance) and right-wing authoritarianism and positively related to innovative behavior and billable hours.[24]	This is the third-generation measure, derived from the original 50-item PVS (see Hardiness Institute, 1985).	Maddi et al. (2006).

54

[23] Vogt et al. (2008) replicate the scale validation using Operation Iraqi Freedom veterans and also find high internal consistency (between .55 and .90), criterion-related validity (i.e., the DRRI was associated with mental and physical health, most strongly with PTSD, depression, and counts of physical symptoms), and discriminate validity (i.e., the DRRI distinguished between men and women and combat and combat support personnel).

[24] In Maddi et al. (2009), the PVS-III-R was shown to be negatively associated with depressive symptoms, anxiety, and hostility but positively associated with avoidance of intrusive, stressful thoughts among a sample of college students. It was also associated with positive attitudes toward school, instructors, and one's own capabilities and standards, as well as life satisfaction.

Name of Measure	Description	Reliability	Validity	Notes	Citation
Brief Resilient Coping Scale (BRCS)	The four-item BRCS captures elements of tenacity, optimism, creativity, an aggressive problem-solving style, and commitment to growth after experiencing difficult situations. It is intended to capture an individual's tendency to cope with stress in an adaptive manner.	Internal consistency ranged from .64 to .76, depending on the survey wave. Test-retest reliability ranged from .68 to .71, depending on the survey wave.	Using a sample of men and women suffering from rheumatoid arthritis, the BRCS was correlated with personal coping resources (e.g., optimism, helplessness, and self-efficacy), pain coping behaviors, and psychological well-being (e.g., positive and negative affect, life satisfaction, and depressive symptoms). Higher scores on the BRCS were associated with lower depressive symptoms but only as levels of stress increased.	Has not seen frequent use in the literature.	Sinclair and Wallston (2004).
Values-in-Action Inventory of Strengths (VIA-IS)	The VIA-IS measures 24 universal character strengths grouped into six domains: wisdom and knowledge, courage, love, justice, temperance, and transcendence.	All subscales had internal consistencies over .70. Test-retest reliability over four months was also over .70 for almost all subscales.	The VIA-IS has been used to differentiate between West Point cadets and the general U.S. population (see Matthews et al., 2006).	The literature search was unable to locate the actual measures.[25] The VIA-IS has been used with *adolescent* samples.	Petersen and Seligman (2004).

---

[25] A list of studies using the VIA-IS can be found at VIA Institute on Character (2015).

Name of Measure	Description	Reliability	Validity	Notes	Citation
Connor-Davidson Resilience Scale (CD-RISC)	The 25-item CD-RISC is drawn from work by Kobasa (1979) on hardiness, Rutter's (1985) work on resiliency, Lyons's (1991) work on enduring stress, and Shackelton's believe in "benevolent intervention" or "good luck." The measure was originally designed to help quantify resilience as a clinical measure to assess treatment response.	Internal consistency of the overall scale was .89. Test-retest reliability was .87. Factor analysis revealed five factors: personal competence, high standards, and tenacity; instincts, tolerance of negative events, and strengthening effects of stress; positive acceptance of change and secure relationships; control; spiritual influences.	The CD-RISC is able to differentiate between clinical and nonclinical samples which are expected to have different levels of resilience.	The CD-RISC is one of the most widely used resilience scales. Has seen some limited use in *adolescent* samples but needs further validation.	Connor and Davidson (2003).
Resilience Scale for Adults (RSA)	The 45-item RSA covers three main categories of resilience: dispositional attributes (e.g., personal competence, social competence, and personal structures), family cohesion/warmth (e.g., family coherence), and external support systems (e.g., social support).	Internal consistency varied by subscale: .90 for personal competence, .83 for social competence, .87 for family coherence, .83 for social support, and .67 for personal structure. Test-retest reliability also varied by subscale: .79 for personal competence, .84 for social competence, .77 for family coherence, .69 for social support, and .74 for personal structure.	The RSA was positively associated with the Sense of Coherence (SOC) scale and negatively correlated with the Hopkins Symptom Check List-25. The scale was also able to discriminate between a clinical and nonclinical community sample.	The RSA was developed using a Norwegian sample. Has seen some limited use in *adolescent* samples but needs further validation.	Friborg et al. (2003).

56

Name of Measure	Description	Reliability	Validity	Notes	Citation
Baruth Protective Factors Inventory (BPFI)	The BPFI is designed to identify the presence of greater resiliency in individuals. The pool of 16 items represents four aspects of resiliency found in prior research: adaptable personality, supportive environment, fewer stressors, and compensating experiences.	Internal consistency varied across the four domains: .76 for adaptive personality, .98 for supportive environment, .55 for fewer stressors, and .83 for compensating experiences. The overall scale alpha was .83.	Several of the domains in the BPFI have been linked to the Multidimensional Health Profile: Psychological Functioning.	The BPFI needs further validation.	Baruth and Carroll (2002).
Resilience Measure [no formal name]	The 11-item measure is based on Kobasa's (1979) definition of hardiness and includes aspects of control, commitment, and change as challenge.	Internal consistency of the overall scale was .73.	Using the National Vietnam Veterans Readjustment Survey, hardiness was directly and negatively associated with PTSD and indirectly associated with PTSD via functional social support.[26]	The literature search was unable to locate the actual measures.	King et al. (1998).
Ego Resilience Scale (ER-89)	The 14-item ER-89 is designed to capture ego-resilience among a general, nonclinical population.	Internal consistency of the overall scale was .76. Test-retest reliability was .67 for women and .51 for men.	Persons high on resiliency tended to be more competent and comfortable in interpersonal relations, as measured by the California Adult Q-Sort.	The original ER-89 was developed in the 1950s. The version used in this study is more recent. "Ego-resiliency" is an older term for resilience, although there are some substantive differences between the two.	Block and Kremen (1996).

[26] The scale has also been used by Taft et al. (1999), Vogt et al. (2008), and King et al. (2006). Vogt et al. report that hardiness in an intermediating factor between combat exposure and PTSD.

Name of Measure	Description	Reliability	Validity	Notes	Citation
Resilience Scale (RS)	The RS is designed to assess an individual's level of resilience, which is viewed by the authors as a positive personality characteristic that enhances individual adaptation. Originally developed from a qualitative study of 24 women who had adapted after a major life event, the 25-item scale represents five dimensions of resilience found in existing literature: equanimity, perseverance, self-reliance, meaningfulness, and existential aloneness.	Internal consistency for the overall scale was .91.[27] Factor analysis yields two factors: personal competence and acceptance of self and life.	Among a random sample of community dwelling older adults (between the ages of 53 and 95) in the Northwest, higher scores on the RS were associated with higher morale, life satisfaction, better self-rated physical health, and lower depression (using the Beck Depression Inventory).	Wagnild (2009) reviewed 12 studies that have used the RS and concluded that it has good internal reliability, instrument validity, and construct validity. However, it is not clear if the RS can be used as an assessment of a resiliency program. The RS has been used with *adolescent* samples.	Wagnild and Young (1993).
Dispositional Resilience Scale (DRS)	The 45-item scale is a modified version of Kobasa's (1979) measure of personality hardiness.[28] In this context, hardiness represents the characteristic manner in which a person approaches and interprets experiences and has three components: commitment, control, and challenge. These components represent the three subscales in the measure.	Internal consistency varied across three subscales from .62 to .85. The overall scale alpha was .85.	Among a sample of 164 Army survivor assistance officers who participated in the Gander air disaster, hardiness was a protective factor. Individuals with high exposure to stress had better health and well-being outcomes (e.g., physical and psychological symptoms, a composite illness index consisting of sick call visits, work days missed, self-rated health, and mood state/happiness) if they also had high levels of hardiness.	Funk's (1992) review of the hardiness literature suggests that the DRS (45-item version) is the most conceptually and psychometrically sound hardiness measure. He cautions that early measures of hardiness are actually capturing neuroticism.	Bartone et al. (1989).

[27] Test-retest reliability reported to be between .67 and .84 among pregnant and postpartum women (Kilien and Jarrett, 1993).

[28] Newer versions of the DRS contain 15 or 30 items (see Bartone 1991, 1995). Bartone (1995, 1999, 2007) reports that the internal consistency of the 15-item version is .82 and established test-retest reliability of .78 over three weeks using a sample of undergraduate freshmen at West Point (see Bartone, 2007).

Table A.2. Measures of Flourishing Among Adults

Name of Measure	Description	Reliability	Validity	Other	Citation
The Flourishing Scale	The Flourishing Scale consists of 8 items describing important aspects of human functioning ranging from positive relationships, to feelings of competence, to having a meaning and purpose in life. High scores indicate that respondents see themselves in a positive light in important areas of functioning. The scale is one-dimensional.	Internal consistency of the overall scale was .87. One-month test-retest reliability was .71. Factor analysis yielded one factor.	The Flourishing Scale was most strongly correlated with competency/mastery and least strongly correlated with autonomy.	The Flourishing Scale is relatively new and has not seen much attention in the literature and needs further validation.	Diener et al. (2010).
Perceived Benefits Scale (PBS)	The 30-item PBS is designed to capture different types of perceived benefits following a stressful event, with the assumption that growth after stress may not occur equally in all domains of life. It has eight subscales: lifestyle changes, material gain, increases in self-efficacy, family closeness, community closeness, faith in people, compassion, and spirituality. Respondents are asked about the event they found most distressing in the past five years.	Internal consistency varied by subscale: Efficacy was .88, community was .85, spirituality was .93, faith in people was .84, compassion was .87, lifestyle was .73, family closeness was .81, and material gain was .74. Two week test-retest reliability also varied by subscale: efficacy was .83, community was .75, spirituality was .93, faith in people was .80, compassion was .66, lifestyle, was .81, family closeness was .85, and material gain was .97.	Means of the subscales did significantly differ depending on the severity of the stressor that was experienced (e.g., death of a loved one, job loss, job stress, divorce, relationship problem, child raising, illness of loved one, and illness of self).		McMillen and Fisher (1998).

Name of Measure	Description	Reliability	Validity	Other	Citation
Thriving Scale	The 20-item Thriving Scale examines a number of social/cultural and personal factors associated with growth after experiencing a stressful event. These factors include appreciation of family, life, and friends, gained positive attitude, personal strength, enhanced spirituality, empathy, and patience. The scale was derived from qualitative interviews with Latina women receiving treatment at a rheumatic disease clinic in New York City, the SRGS, and the PTGI (see below).	Internal consistency for the overall scale was .92.	Thriving was associated with competence, as measured by self-esteem and self-efficacy, and psychological well-being, as measured by positive and negative affect.	The Thriving Scale has not seen much attention in the literature. The validation sample is very specialized and small. All questions are introduced with "Because of my illness…" so it is not clear how well the measure would work for other stressful events or conditions.	Abraído-Lanza, Guier, and Colón (1998).
Post-Traumatic Growth Inventory (PTGI)	The 21-item PTGI is designed to capture positive outcomes reported by persons who have experienced traumatic events. It includes five factors: new possibilities, relating to others, personal strength, spiritual change, and appreciation for life. Scale items refer to respondents' self-reported stressful events experienced in the past five years although any time frame can be used.	Internal consistency for the overall scale was .90. Internal consistency varied by domain: New possibilities was .84, relating to others was .85, personal strength .85, spiritual change was .72, appreciation of life was .67. Test-retest reliability over two months was .71.	The PTGI was modestly (.16 to .29) and positively correlated with optimism, extraversion, openness, agreeableness, and conscientious (but not neuroticism) as measured by the Neuroticism-Extraversion-Openness personality inventory. It was also modestly, positively correlated with religious participation (.25). Respondents who reported severe trauma over the past year scored significantly higher on the PTGI than those who did not. This was also true of the subscales with the exception of the spiritual change factor.	The PTGI has been adapted by several authors for use in *child and adolescent* samples (see below).	Tedeschi and Calhoun (1996).

60

Name of Measure	Description	Reliability	Validity	Other	Citation
Stress-Related Growth Scale (SRGS)	The 50-item SRGS is designed to measure self-reported positive outcomes following a stressful event. Scale items are completed with respect to the respondent's most stressful event in the past year, although this time frame is flexible. The SRGS is a unidimensional scale and measures only positive growth.	Internal consistency for the overall scale was .94. Two-week test-retest for a subsample was .81.	Intrinsic religiousness (the degree to which religion serves as a framework for meaning), social support satisfaction, stressfulness of the negative event, positive reinterpretation and acceptance of coping, and number of recent positive events were all significant predictors of the SRGS. Using longitudinal data, the SRGS was positively associated with change in optimism, positive affect, number of socially supportive others, and social support satisfaction after experiencing a self-reported negative event.	The SRGS has seen the most use in the research literature.[29] Results of validation study using college students may be due to maturation rather than positive growth after experiencing stress.	Park Cohen, and Murch (1996).

[29] Armeli, Gunthert, and Cohen (2001) propose a revised version of the SRGS that includes 43 of the original 50 items (seven items could not be neutrally reworded and thus were dropped). In the revised version, items are reworded to allow for either positive or negative growth following a stressful event. This revised measure yielded seven factors: treatment of others, religiousness, personal strength, belongingness, affect-regulation, self-understanding, and optimism. Internal consistency ranged by subscale from .67 to .90 among an adult sample and .61 to .87 among a college student sample. Results of this work suggest that post-stress growth is most likely to occur when individuals (1) experience a very highly stressful event, (2) have high levels of pre-event personal and social resources, and (3) use adaptive coping strategies.

61

Name of Measure	Description	Reliability	Validity	Other	Citation
Changes in Outlook Questionnaire	The 26-item Changes in Outlook Questionnaire is designed to assess both positive and negative changes in an individual's outlook on life following a traumatic event. The measure was developed from responses to an open-ended question about the ways in which a trauma survivor's life view/outlook had changed following the event (this was dissertation work done by the first author). Only items that were rated as unambiguously positive or unambiguously negative by five psychology raters are included in the measure.	Internal consistency for the positive response subscale was .83 and included 11 items. The internal consistency for the negative response subscale was .90 and included 15 items.	Using a small sample of trauma survivors, higher scores on the negative response scale were found to correlate with other measures of post-traumatic symptomatology (i.e., the General Health Questionnaire, anxiety and insomnia, and depression), maladaptive coping style (i.e., lower self-esteem, weaker world beliefs, and more internal responsibility for negative outcomes), and reduced social support. No associations were found for the positive response subscale.	The validation sample was very small (n = 35). Further, it is not clear if the measure will stand up within a sample where levels of trauma vary.	Joseph, Williams, and Yule (1993).

62

Table A.3. Measures of Resilience and Hardiness Among Children and Adolescents

Name of Measure	Description	Reliability	Validity	Other	Citation
ClassMaps Survey (CMS)	CMS is designed to measure aspects of classrooms that promote resiliency among students. It contains seven subscales and 47 measures.[30] Four subscales describe relations aspects of the classroom: teacher-student relationships, peer friendships, peer conflict, and home-school relationships. Three subscales describe autonomy-promoting characteristics: academic self-efficacy, self-determination, and behavior self-control.	Internal consistency varied across subscales, from .82 to .91.	The CMS subscales were positively associated with the Student Engagement in Science scale, the Efficacy for Science Inquiry scale, the Value of Science scale (VS), and the Science Career Interest scale. The self-efficacy, self-determination, and teacher-student subscales were most strongly associated with the validation measures.	The current study was the first to use the CMS in a middle school sample.[31] Has not seen frequent use in the literature.	Doll et al. (2010).
Devereux Early Childhood Assessment Clinical Form (DECA-C)	The 62-item DECA-C is intended to measure resilience in preschoolers from ages 2 to 5 with social and emotional problems or significant behavioral concerns.[32] It is standardized and norm-referenced and is part of a larger DECA program. It includes three protective factor subscales (initiative, self-control, and attachment) in adaption to four behavioral concern scales (attention problems, aggression, withdrawal/depression, and emotional control problems). The Total Behavioral Concerns Scale is a composite of the four behavioral concerns scales.	Internal consistency varied across subscales: .66 (withdrawal/ depression) to .78 (emotional control problems for parents) and .80 (withdrawal/ depression) to .90 (attention problems for teachers).	The DECA-C was able to differentiate between a clinical and community sample with 74 percent accuracy.	The DECA-C can be completed by both teachers and parents but must be interpreted by a behavioral healthcare or special education professional. Has not seen frequent use in the literature.	LeBuffe, Shapiro, and Naglieri (2009).

---

[30] An additional subscale that measures bullying and aggressive behavior was omitted from this study because science teachers deemed it not relevant.

[31] See also Doll and Siemers (2004), Doll, Zucker, and Brehm (2004), and Doll et al. (2009). These studies examined psychometric properties of the CMS using samples of elementary aged students. Internal consistency ranged from .78 to .93.

[32] The DECA-C is described in more detail in LeBuffe and Naglieri (2003) (see also LeBuffe, Shapiro, and Naglieri, 2009).

Name of Measure	Description	Reliability	Validity	Other	Citation
Resiliency Scales for Adolescents (RSCA)	The 64-item RCSA assesses resiliency in normal populations for the purpose of screening and preventive interventions for at-risk children and adolescents. It contains three self-report scales, which themselves comprise 10 constructs: sense of mastery, sense of relatedness, and emotional reactivity. In additional, two index scores measure resources and vulnerability.	Internal consistency ranged from .85 to .97 depending on subscale and age group in a community sample. In clinical samples, internal consistency ranged from .44 to .91 among 9- to 14-year-olds and .81 to .96 for 15- to 18-year-olds.	Findings suggest that the RCSA can be used in clinical samples to examine dimensions of normative development.	Scores are normed for three age groups: 9 to 11, 12 to 14, and 15 to 18. Technical manuals can be found in Prince-Embury (2006, 2007).[33]	Prince-Embury (2010).
Adolescent Resiliency Scale (ARS)	The 21-item ARS consists of three factor subscales: novelty-seeking, emotional regulation, and positive future orientation.	Internal consistency ranged by subscale: .79 for novelty seeking. .77 for emotional regulation, and .81 for future orientation. The internal consistency for the overall scale was .85.	The ARS was able to distinguish between well-adjusted and resilient groups and a vulnerable group.[34]	The ARS was developed using a Japanese sample. Has not been seen frequent use in the literature.	Oshio et al. (2003).

---

[33] See also Prince-Embury and Steer (2010).

[34] Using the General Health Questionnaire and a list of negative life events, Oshio et al. (2003) created three subgroups in their sample of Japanese undergraduates: well adjusted (i.e., mentally healthy with few life events), vulnerable (i.e., poorer mental health with many negative life events), and resilient (i.e., healthy despite many negative life events).

Name of Measure	Description	Reliability	Validity	Other	Citation
Resiliency Attitudes and Scales Profile (RASP)	The 34-item RASP is intended to measure resiliency among youth for recreation and other social services. It is targeted at at-risk populations; however, it should not be used as a diagnostic tool. It contains seven dimensions: insight, independence, creativity, humor, initiative, relationships, and value orientation.	Internal consistency varied by subscale: .65 for insight, .62 for independence, .68 for creativity, .49 for humor, .71 for relationships, .53 for initiative, and .68 for value orientation. The internal consistency for the overall scale was .91. Five-day test-retest reliability was .94.	Scores on the RASP were positively associated with psychosocial well-being and negatively associated with psychological distress as measured by the Mental Health Inventory.	May be best used as a program evaluation tool to see if a resilience program has improved overall group resilience. Has not seen frequent use in the literature.	Hurtes and Allen (2001).
Resilience as a Belief System (RBS)	The 37-item RBS contains four subscales: optimism, future orientation, belief in others, and independence.	Internal consistency varied by subscale: .82 for optimism, .70 for future orientation, .66 for belief in others, and .66 for independence. Test-retest reliability also varied by subscale: .68 for optimism, .58 for future orientation, .58 for belief in others, and .70 for independence.	The RBS was able to differentiate between a clinical and community sample.	Independence subscale appears to be most problematic.	Jew, Green, and Kroger (1999).

Table A.4. Measures of Flourishing Among Children and Adolescents[35]

Name of Measure	Description	Reliability	Validity	Other	Citation
Posttraumatic Growth Measure (PTG)	This adaptation of the PTGI measures the degree to which change occurred in a person's life as a result of a significant event. On the basis of a pilot test with 20 adolescent girls, the authors altered the original PTGI in three ways: (1) some items were reworded to enhance comprehension among the younger sample, (2) the response scale was truncated to three (i.e., no change, a little change, a lot of change), and (3) the factor representing spiritual change was dropped leaving four subscales (i.e., appreciation of life, relating to others, personal strength, and new possibilities).	Internal consistency for the overall scale was .90. Internal consistency varied by subscale, from .72 to .80.	Different types of stressful events were associated with different PTG profiles based on the four subscales (e.g., interpersonal problems resulted in lower levels of growth on the "appreciation of life" subscale compared to pregnancy and motherhood or death of a loved one). Controlling for baseline emotional distress, PTG was associated with subsequent reduction in short- and long-term emotional distress.	The sample consists only of low socio-economic, inner city female adolescents.	Ickovics et al. (2006).
Posttraumatic Growth Inventory for Children (PTGI-C)	The 21-item PTGI-C is an adaptation of the original PTGI for use in adolescent samples. It contains five domains: new possibilities, relating to others, personal strength, appreciation of life, and spiritual change. The scale measures only positive growth.	Internal consistency for the overall scale is .89.	Competency beliefs were positively and significantly associated with the PTGI-C. Self-reporting of rumination was not significantly associated with PTG. Social support may be indirectly associated with PTG via competency beliefs.		Cryder et al. (2006).

---

[35] For a recent review of post-traumatic growth in youth and adolescents see Clay, Knibbs, and Joseph (2009).

66

Name of Measure	Description	Reliability	Validity	Other	Citation
Posttraumatic Growth Measure	This measure contains 16 items adapted from the original PTGI for adults as well as new measures created by the first author. PTG is assessed with respect to a self-nominated stressful event that could have occurred at any point in the past (adolescents are asked how long ago the event occurred). The measure is designed to capture both positive and negative changes in response to stress.	Internal consistency for the overall scale was .93.	Older adolescents reported higher levels of PTG; however, this may attributable to higher levels of maturity. High PTG scores were associated with lower substance use but were not associated with depression or religiosity after controls were included.	This adaptation of the PTGI has not seen much attention in the literature.	Milam, Ritt-Olson, and Unger (2004).
Posttraumatic Growth Inventory— Revised for Children and Adolescents	This adaptation of the *PTGI* contains 21 reworded items suitable for children as young as age 8.	Internal consistency for the overall scale was .94. Internal consistency also varied by subscale, ranging from .68 to .86.	No difference was found between parents' and children's self-reported ratings of PTG. Total social support was a predictor of PTG whereas self-efficacy and parents' report of PTG were not.	This is a doctoral dissertation and this adaptation of the PTGI has not seen much attention in the literature.	Yaskowich (2002).

References

Abraído-Lanza, A. F., C. Guier, and R. M. Colón, "Psychological Thriving Among Latinas with Chronic Illness," *Journal of Social Issues*, Vol. 54, 1998, pp. 405–524.

Almedom, A. M., "Resilience, Hardiness, Sense of Coherence, and Post-traumatic Growth: All Paths Leading to 'Light at the End of the Tunnel'," *Journal of Loss and Trauma*, Vol. 10, 2005, pp. 253–265.

Antonovsky, A., "The Structure and Properties of the Sense of Coherence Scale," *Social Science and Medicine*, Vol. 36, 1993, pp. 725–733.

Antonovsky, H., and S. Sagy, "The Development of a Sense of Coherence and Its Impact on Responses to Stress Situations," *Journal of Social Psychology*, Vol. 126, 1986, pp. 213–225.

Armeli, S., K. C. Gunthert, and L. H. Cohen, "Stressor Appraisals, Coping, and Post-Event Outcomes: The Dimensionality and Antecedents of Stress-related Growth," *Journal of Social and Clinical Psychology*, Vol. 20, 2001, pp. 366–395.

Baruth, K. E., and J. J. Carroll, "A Formal Assessment of Resilience: The Baruth Protective Factors Inventory," *Journal of Individual Psychology*, Vol. 58, 2002, pp. 235–244.

Bartone, P. T., "Test-Retest Reliability of the Dispositional Resilience Scale-15, a Brief Hardiness Scale," *Psychological Reports*, Vol. 101, 2007, pp. 934–944.

——— "Resilience Under Military Operational Stress: Can Leaders Influence Hardiness?" *Military Psychology,* Vol. 18, 2006, pp. S131–S148.

——— "Hardiness Protects Against War-related Stress in Army Reserve Forces," *Consulting Psychology Journal*, Vol. 51, 1999, pp. 72–82.

——— "A Short Hardiness Scale," paper presented at the American Psychological Society Convention, New York, 1995.

——— "Development and Validation of a Short Hardiness Measure," paper presented at the Annual Convention of the American Psychological Society, Washington, D.C., 1991.

Bartone, P. T., R. J. Ursano, K. M. Wright, and L. H. Ingraham, "The Impact of a Military Air Disaster on the Health of Assistance Workers," *Journal of Nervous and Mental Disease*, Vol. 177, 1989, pp. 317–328.

Bates, M. J., S. Bowles, J. Hammermeister, C. Stokes, E. Pinder, M. Moore, M. Fritts, M. Vythilingam, T. Yosick, J. Rhodes, C. Myatt, R. Westphal, D. Fautua, P. Hammer, and

G. Burbelo, "Psychological Fitness," *Military Medicine,* Vol. 175 (Supplement), 2010, pp. 21–38.

Bishop, G. D., D. Kaur, V. L. Tan, Y. L. Chua, S. M. Liew, and K. H. Mak, "Effects of a Psychosocial Skills Training Workshop on Psychophysiological and Psychosocial Risk in Patients Undergoing Coronary Artery Bypass Grafting," *American Heart Journal*, Vol. 150, 2005, pp. 602–609.

Block, J., and A. M. Kremen, "IQ and Ego-Resiliency: Conceptual and Empirical Connections and Separateness," *Journal of Personality and Social Psychology*, Vol. 70, 1996, pp. 349–361.

Bonanno, G. A., "Resilience in the Face of Potential Trauma," *Current Directions in Psychological Science*, Vol. 14, No.3, 2005, pp. 135–138.

Bonanno, G. A., M. Westphal, and A. D. Mancini, "Resilience to Loss and Potential Trauma," *Annual Review of Clinical Psychology*, Vol. 7, 2011, pp. 511–535.

Bray, R. M., J. L. Spira, K. R. Olmsted, and J. J. Hout, "Behavioral and Occupational Fitness," *Military Medicine,* Vol. 175 (Supplement 1), 2010, pp. 39–56.

Brierley-Bowers, P., S. Sexton, D. Brown, and M. Bates, *Measures of Autonomic Nervous System Regulation*, Arlington, Va.: Defense Centers of Excellence for Psychological Health and Traumatic Brain Injury (DCoE), April 2011.

Brunwasser, S. M., J. E. Gillham, and E. S. Kim, "A Meta-Analytic Review of the Penn Resiliency Program's Effect on Depressive Symptoms," *Journal of Consulting and Clinical Psychology*, Vol. 77, 2009, pp. 1042–1054.

Cacioppo, J. T., H. T. Reis, and A. J. Zautra, "The Value of Social Fitness with an Application to the Military," *American Psychologist*, Vol. 66, 2011, pp. 43–51.

Carver, C. S., "Resilience and Thriving: Issues, Models, and Linkages," *Journal of Social Issues*, Vol. 54, No. 2, 1998, pp. 245–266.

Chrousos, G. P., "Stressors, Stress, and Neuroendocrine Integration of the Adaptive Response: The 1997 Hans Selye Memorial Lecture," *Annals of the New York Academy of Science*, Vol. 851, 1998, pp. 311–335.

Clay, R., J. Knibbs, and S. Joseph, "Measurement of Post-Traumatic Growth in Young People: A Review," *Clinical Child Psychology and Psychiatry*, Vol. 14, 2009, pp. 411–422.

Connor, K. M., and J. R. T. Davidson, "Development of a New Resilience Scale: The Connor-Davidson Resilience Scale (CD-RISC)," *Depression and Anxiety*, Vol. 18, 2003, pp. 76–82.

Cornum, R., and P. Copeland, *She Went to War: The Rhonda Cornum Story*, Novato, Calif.: Presidio Press, 1993.

Coulter, I., P. Lester, and J. Yarvis, "Social Fitness," *Military Medicine*, Vol. 175, No. 8S, 2010, pp. 88–96.

Cryder, C. H., M. A. Ryan, R. P. Kilmer, R. G. Tedeschi, and L. Calhoun, "An Exploratory Study of Post-Traumatic Growth in Children Following a Natural Disaster," *American Journal of Orthopsychiatry*, Vol. 76, 2006, pp. 65–69.

Davidson, K. W., Y. Gidron, E. Mostofsky, and K. J. Trudeau, "Hospitalization Cost Offset of a Hostility Intervention for Coronary Heart Disease Patients," *Journal of Consulting and Clinical Psychology*, Vol. 75, 2007, pp. 657–662.

Defense Centers of Excellence for Psychological Health and Traumatic Brain Injury (DCoE), *Traumatic Brain Injury*, 2011. As of April 9, 2011:
http://www.dcoe.health.mil/TraumaticBrainInjury.aspx

Department of the Navy, *Combat and Operational Stress Control* (NTTP 1-15M), Washington D.C., 2010.

Diener, E., D. Wirtz, W. Tov, C. Kim-Prieto, D. Choi, S. Oishi, and R. Biswas-Diener, "New Well-Being Measures: Short Scales to Assess Flourishing and Positive and Negative Feelings," *Social Indicators Research*, Vol. 97, 2010, pp. 143–156.

Dolan, C. A., and A. B. Adler, "Military Hardiness as a Buffer of Psychological Health on Return from Deployment," *Military Medicine*, Vol. 171, 2006, pp. 93–98.

Doll, B., and E. Siemers, "Assessing Instructional Climate: The Reliability and Validity of ClassMaps," poster session presented at the Annual Convention of the National Association of School Psychologists, Dallas, Tex., 2004a.

Doll, B., S. Zucker, and K. Brehm, *Resilient Classrooms: Creating Healthier Environments for Learning*, New York: Guilford Press, 2004b.

Doll, B., S. Curien, C. LeClair, R. Spies, A. Chamption, and A. Osborn, "The ClassMaps Survey: A Framework for Promoting Positive Classroom Environments," in R. Gilman, S. Huebner, and M. Furlong (Eds.,), *Handbook of Positive Psychology in the Schools*, New York: Routledge, 2009, pp. 213–227.

Doll, B., R. A. Spies, A. Champion, C. Guerrero, K. Dooley, and A. Turner, "The ClassMaps Survey: A Measure of Middle School Science Students' Perceptions of Classroom Characteristics," *Journal of Psychological Assessment*, Vol. 28, 2010, pp. 338–348.

Eriksson, M., and B. Lindström, "Antonovsky's Sense of Coherence Scale and the Relation with Health: A Systematic Review," *Journal of Epidemiology and Community Health*, Vol. 60, 2006, pp. 376–381.

Eschleman, K. J., N. A. Bowling, and G. M. Alarcon, "A Meta-analytic Examination of Hardiness," *International Journal of Stress Management*, Vol. 17, 2010, pp. 277–307.

Fikretoglu, D., A. Brunet, J. Poundja, S. Guay, and D. Pedlar, "Validation of the Deployment Risk and Resilience Inventory in French-Canadian Veterans: Findings on the Relation Between Deployment Experiences and Post-Deployment Health," *Canadian Journal of Psychiatry*, Vol. 51, 2006, pp. 755–763.

Flórez, K. R., R. A. Shih, and M. T. Martin, *Nutritional Fitness and Resilience: A Review of Relevant Constructs, Measures, and Links to Well-Being*, Santa Monica, Calif.: RAND Corporation, RR-105-AF, 2014. As of January 28, 2013:
http://www.rand.org/pubs/research_reports/RR105.html

Friborg, O., O. Hjemdal, J. H. Rosenvinge, and M. Martinussen, "A New Rating Scale for Adult Resilience: What Are the Central Protective Resources Behind Healthy Adjustment?" *International Journal of Methods in Psychiatric Research*, Vol. 12, 2003, pp. 65–76.

Funk, S. C., "Hardiness: A Review of Theory and Research," *Health Psychology*, Vol. 11, 1992, pp. 335–345.

Gidron, Y., K. Davidson, and I. Bata, "The Short-Term Effects of a Hostility-Reduction Intervention on Male Coronary Heart Disease Patients," *Health Psychology*, Vol. 18, 1999, pp. 416–420.

Hardiness Institute, *Personal Views Survey*, Arlington Heights, Il., 1985.

Hobfoll, S. E., "Conservation of Resources: A New Attempt at Conceptualizing Stress," *American Psychologist,* Vol. 44, No. 3, 1989, pp. 513–524.

Hobfoll, S. E., "Conservation of Resources Theory: Its Implication for Stress, Health and Resilience, in S. Folkman (Ed.), *Handbook of Stress, Health and Coping,* New York: Oxford University Press, 2011, pp. 127–147.

Horowitz, J. L., and J. Garber, "The Prevention of Depressive Symptoms in Children and Adolescents: A Meta-analytic Review," *Journal of Consulting and Clinical Psychology*, Vol. 74, 2006, pp. 401–415.

Hurtes, K. P., and L. R. Allen, "Measuring Resiliency in Youth: The Resiliency Attitudes and Skills Profile," *Therapeutic Recreation Journal*, Vol. 35, 2010, pp. 333–347.

Ickovics, J. R., C. S. Mede, T. S. Kershaw, S. Milan, J. B. Lewis, and K. A. Ethier, "Urban Teens: Trauma, Post-traumatic Growth, and Emotional Distress Among Female Adolescents," *Journal of Consulting and Clinical Psychology*, Vol. 74, 2006, pp. 841–850.

Jensen, P. S., R. L. Lewis, and S. N. Xenakis, "The Military Family in Review: Context, Risk, and Prevention," *Journal of the American Academy of Child Psychiatry*, Vol. 25, 1986, pp. 225–234.

Jew, C. L., K. E. Green, and J. Kroger, "Development and Validation of a Measure of Resilience," *Measurement and Evaluation in Counseling and Development*, Vol. 32, 1999, pp. 75–89.

Johnson, D. C., M. A. Polusny, C. R. Erbes, D. King, L. King, B. T. Litz, P. P. Schurr, M. Friedman, R. H. Pietrak, and S. M. Southwick, "Development and Initial Validation of the Response to Stressful Experiences Scale," *Military Medicine*, Vol. 176, 2011, pp. 161–169.

Joseph, S., R. Williams, and W. Yule, "Changes in Outlook Following a Disaster: The Preliminary Development of a Measure to Assess Positive and Negative Responses," *Journal of Traumatic Stress*, Vol. 6, 1993, pp. 271–279.

Judkins, S., et al., "Hardiness Training Among Nurse Managers: Building a Healthy Workplace," *Journal of Continuing Education in Nursing*, Vol. 37, 2006, pp. 202–207.

Kemeny, M. E., "The Psychobiology of Stress," *Current Directions in Psychological Science*, Vol. 12, 2003, pp. 124–129.

Keyes, C. L. M., "The Mental Health Continuum: From Languishing to Flourishing in Life," *Journal of Health and Social Behavior*, Vol. 43, 2002, pp. 207–222.

Kilien, M., and M. E. Jarrett, "Returning to Work: Impact on Postpartum Mothers Health," unpublished raw data, cited in G. M. Wagnild and H. M. Young, "Development and Psychometric Evaluation of the Resilience Scale," *Journal of Nursing Measurement*, Vol. 1, 1993, pp. 165–178.

King, L. A., D. W. King, J. A. Fairbank, T. M. Keane, and G. A. Adams, "Resilience-Recovery Factors in Post-Traumatic Stress Disorder Among Male and Female Vietnam Veterans: Hardiness, Post-War Social Support, and Additional Stressful Life Events," *Journal of Personality and Social Psychology*, Vol. 74, 1998, pp. 420–434.

King, L. A., D. W. King, D. S. Vogt, J. Knight, and R. E. Samper, "Deployment Risk and Resilience Inventory: A Collection of Measures for Studying Deployment-Related Experiences of Military Personnel and Veterans," *Military Psychology*, Vol. 18, 2006, pp. 89–120.

Kirby, E. D., V. P. Williams, M. C. Hocking, J. D. Lane, and R. B. Williams, "Psychosocial Benefits of Three Formats of a Standardized Behavioral Stress Management Program," *Psychosomatic Medicine*, Vol. 68, 2006, pp. 816–823.

Kobasa, S. C., "Stressful Life Events, Personality, and Health: An Inquiry into Hardiness," *Journal of Personality and Social Psychology*, Vol. 37, No. 1, 1979, pp. 1–11.

Kobasa, S. C., and S. R. Maddi, "Existential Personality Theory," in R. J. Corsini (Ed.), *Current Personality Theories*, Chicago: Peacock, 1977, pp. 243–276.

Kuehn, B. H., "Soldier Suicide Rates Continue to Rise: Military, Scientists Work to Stem the Tide," *Journal of the American Medical Association,* Vol. 301, 2009, pp. 1111–1113.

LeBuffe, P.A., and J. A. Naglieri, *The Devereux Early Childhood Assessment Clinical Form (DECA-C): A Measure of Behaviors Related to Risk and Resilience in Preschool Children*, Lewisville, N.C.: Kaplan Press, 2003.

LeBuffe, P.A., V. B. Shapiro, and J. A. Naglieri, *The Devereux Student Strengths Assessment (DESSA)*, Lewisville, N.C.: Kaplan Press, 2009.

Lester, P. B., P. D. Harms, M. N. Herian, D. V. Krasikova, and S. J. Beal, *The Comprehensive Soldier Fitness Program Evaluation Report #3: Longitudinal Analysis of the Impact of Master Resilience Training on Self-Reported Resilience and Psychological Health Data*, United States Army, 2011.

Lyons, J., "Strategies for Assessing the Potential for Positive Adjustment Following Trauma," *Journal of Traumatic Stress*, Vol. 4, 1991, pp. 93–111.

Maddi, S. R., "Relevance of Hardiness Assessment and Training to the Military Context," *Military Psychology*, Vol. 19, 2007, pp. 61–70.

——— "The Story of Hardiness: Twenty Years of Theorizing, Research, and Practice," *Consulting Psychology Journal: Practice and Research*, Vol. 54, 2002, pp. 173–185.

Maddi, S. R., et al., "Hardiness Training Facilitates Performance in College," *Journal of Positive Psychology*, Vol. 4, 2009, pp. 566–577.

Maddi, S. R., R. H. Harvey, D. M. Khoshaba, J. L. Lu, M. Persico, and M. Brow, "The Personality Construct of Hardiness, III: Innovativeness, Authoritarianism, and Performance," *Journal of Personality*, Vol. 74, 2006, pp. 575–597.

Maddi, S. R., S. Kahn, and K. L. Maddi, "The Effectiveness of Hardiness Training," *Consulting Psychology Journal: Practice and Research*, Vol. 50, 1998, pp. 78–86.

Madsen, M. D., and N. Abell, "Trauma Resilience Scale: Validation of Protective Factors Associated with Adaptation Following Violence," *Research on Social Work Practice*, Vol. 20, 2010, pp. 223–233.

Masten, A., and J. Obradovic, "Competence and Resilience in Development," *Annals of the New York Academy of Science*, Vol. 1094, 2006, pp. 13–27.

McEwen, B. S, and E. Stellar, "Stress and the Individual: Mechanisms Leading to Disease," *Archives of Internal Medicine*, Vol. 153, No. 18, 1993, pp. 2093–2101.

McGene, J., *Social Fitness and Resilience: A Review of Relevant Constructs, Measures, and Links to Well-Being.* Santa Monica, Calif.: RAND Corporation, RR-108-AF, 2013. As of January 28, 2013:
http://www.rand.org/pubs/research_reports/RR108.html

Meredith, L. S., C. D. Sherbourne, S. Gaillot, L. Hansell, H. V. Ritschard, A. M. Parker, and G. Wrenn, *Promoting Psychological Resilience in the U.S. Military,* Santa Monica, Calif.: RAND Corporation, MG-996-OSD, 2011. As of May 24, 2015:
http://www.rand.org/pubs/monographs/MG996.html

McMillen, J. C., and R. H. Fisher, "The Perceived Benefits Scale: Measuring Positive Life Changes After Negative Events," *Social Work Research*, Vol. 22, 1998, pp. 173–186.

Milam, J. E., A. Ritt-Olson, and J. Unger, "Post-Traumatic Growth Among Adolescents," *Journal of Adolescent Research*, Vol. 19, 2004, pp. 192–203.

Mullen, A. M., "On Total Force Fitness in War and Peace," *Military Medicine*, Vol. 175 (Supplement), 2010, pp. 1–2.

O'Leary, V. E., and J. R. Ickovics, "Resilience and Thriving in Response to Challenge: An Opportunity for a Paradigm Shift in Women's Health," *Women's Health: Research on Gender, Behavior, and Policy*, Vol. 1, 1995, pp. 121–142.

Oshio, A., H. Kaneko, S. Nagamine, and M. Nakaya, "Construct Validity of the Adolescent Resiliency Scale," *Psychological Reports*, Vol. 93, 2003, pp. 1217–1222.

Park, C. L., L. H. Cohen, and R. L. Murch, "Assessment and Prediction of Stress-Related Growth," *Journal of Personality*, Vol. 64, 1996, pp. 72–105.

Pearlin, L. I., E. G. Menaghan, M. A. Lieberman, and J. T. Mullan, "The Stress Process," *Journal of Health and Social Behavior*, Vol. 22, No. 4, 1981, pp. 337–356.

Petersen, C., and M. E. P. Seligman, *Character Strengths and Virtues: A Handbook and Classification*, New York: Oxford, 2004.

Polk, L. V., "Toward a Middle-Range Theory of Resilience," A*dvances in Nursing Science*, Vol. 19, No. 3, 1997, pp. 1–13.

Prince-Embury, S., "Psychometric Properties of the Resiliency Scales for Adolescents and Use for Youth with Psychiatric Disorders," *Journal of Psychoeducational Assessment*, Vol. 28, 2010, pp. 291–302.

———— *Resiliency Scales for Adolescents: Profiles of Personal Strengths*, San Antonio, Tex.: Harcourt Assessments, 2007.

———— *Resiliency Scales for Children and Adolescents: Profiles of Personal Strengths*, San Antonio, Tex.: Harcourt Assessments, 2006.

Prince-Embury, S., and R. Steer, "Profiles of Personal Resiliency as Assessed by the Resiliency Scales for Children and Adolescents," *Journal of Psychoeducational Assessment*, Vol. 28, 2010, pp. 303–314.

Ramchand, R., J. Acosta, R. M. Burns, L. H. Jaycox, and C. G. Pernin, *The War Within: Preventing Suicide in the U.S. Military*, Santa Monica, Calif.: RAND Corporation, MG-953-OSD, 2011. As of April 9, 2011:
http://www.rand.org/pubs/monographs/MG953

Richardson, G. E., "The Metatheory of Resilience and Resiliency," *Journal of Clinical Psychology*, Vol. 58, No. 3, 2002, pp. 307–321.

Robson, S., *Physical Fitness and Resilience: A Review of Relevant Constructs, Measures, and Links to Well-Being.* Santa Monica, Calif.: RAND Corporation, RR-104-AF, 2013. As of January 28, 2013:
http://www.rand.org/pubs/research_reports/RR104.html

———, *Psychological Fitness and Resilience: A Review of Relevant Constructs, Measures, and Links to Well-Being.* Santa Monica, Calif.: RAND Corporation, RR-102-AF, 2014. As of January 28, 2013:
http://www.rand.org/pubs/research_reports/RR102.html

Robson, S., and N. Salcedo, *Behavioral Fitness and Resilience: A Review of Relevant Constructs, Measures, and Links to Well-Being.* Santa Monica, Calif.: RAND Corporation, RR-103-AF, 2014. As of September 11, 2015:
http://www.rand.org/pubs/research_reports/RR103.html

Rosen, Leora N., and D. B. Durand, "Marital Adjustment Following Deployment," in James A. Martin, Leora N. Rosen, and Linette R. Sparacino (Eds.), *The Military Family: A Practice Guide for Human Service Providers*, Westport, Conn.: Praeger, 2000, pp. 153–165.

Rutter, M., "Resilience, Competence and Coping," *Child Abuse and Neglect*, Vol. 31, 2007, pp. 205–209.

——— "Psychosocial Resilience and Protective Mechanisms," *American Journal of Orthopsychiatry*, Vol. 57, No. 3, 1987, pp. 316–331.

——— "Resilience in the Face of Adversity: Protective Factors to Resistance to Psychiatric Disorder," *British Journal of Psychiatry*, Vol. 147, 1985, pp. 598–611.

Sayers, S. L., "Family Reintegration Difficulties and Couples Therapy for Military Veterans and Their Spouses," *Cognitive and Behavioral Practice*, Vol. 18, 2011, pp. 108–119.

Segal, M. W., "The Military and the Family as Greedy Institutions," *Armed Forces & Society*, Vol. 13, 1986, pp. 9–38.

Seligman, M. E. P., "Building Resilience," *Harvard Business Review,* April 2011, pp. 101–106.

Seligman, M. E. P., and M. Csikszentmihalyi, "Positive Psychology: An Introduction," *American Psychologist*, Vol. 55, 2000. pp. 5–14.

Selye, H., "Stress and the General Adaptation Syndrome," *British Medical Journal*, Vol. 1, No. 4667, 1950, pp. 1383–1392.

——— "On the Real Benefits of Eustress," *Psychology Today*, Vol. 12, 1978, pp. 60–64.

Shih, R. A., S. O. Meadows, and M. T. Martin, *Medical Fitness and Resilience: A Review of Relevant Constructs, Measures, and Links to Well-Being,* Santa Monica, Calif.: RAND Corporation, RR-107-AF, 2013. As of January 28, 2013: http://www.rand.org/pubs/research_reports/RR107.html

Shih, R., S. O. Meadows, J. M. Mendeloff, and K. Bowling, *Environmental Fitness and Resilience: A Review of Relevant Constructs, Measures, and Links to Well-Being,* Santa Monica, Calif.: RAND Corporation, RR-101-AF, 2015. As of October 2015: http://www.rand.org/pubs/research_reports/RR101.html

Simmons, A., and L. Yoder, "Military Resilience: A Concept Analysis," *Nursing Forum,* Vol. 48, No. 1, 2013, pp. 17–25.

Sinclair, V. G., and K. A. Wallston, "The Development and Psychometric Evaluation of a Brief Resilient Coping Scale," *Assessment*, Vol. 11, 2004, pp. 94–110.

Skomorovsky, A., and K. A. Sudom, "Role of Hardiness in the Psychological Well-Being of Canadian Forces Officer Candidates," *Military Medicine*, Vol. 176, 2011, pp. 7–12.

Smith, B. W., J. Dalen, K. Wiggins, E. Tooley, P. Christopher, and J. Bernard, "The Brief Resilience Scale: Assessing the Ability to Bounce Back," *International Journal of Behavioral Medicine*, Vol. 15, 2008, pp. 194–200.

Smith, S. L., "Could Comprehensive Soldier Fitness Have Iatrogenic Consequences? A Commentary," *The Journal of Behavioral Health Services & Research,* 2013, Vol. 40, No. 2, pp. 242–246.

Steenkamp, M. M., W. P. Nash, and B. T. Litz, "Post-Traumatic Stress Disorder: Review of Comprehensive Soldier Fitness Program," *American Journal of Preventive Medicine,* Vol. 44, No. 5, 2013, pp. 507–512.

Stice, E., H. Shaw, C. Bohon, C. N. Marti, and P. Rohde, "A Meta-Analytic Review of Depression Prevention Programs for Children and Adolescents: Factors That Predict Magnitude of Intervention Effects," *Journal of Consulting and Clinical Psychology*, Vol. 77, 2009, pp. 486–503.

Tanielian, T., and L. Jaycox (Eds.), *Invisible Wounds of War: Psychological and Cognitive Injuries, Their Consequences, and Services to Assist Recovery*, Santa Monica, Calif.: RAND Corporation, MG-720-CCF, 2008. As of May 24, 2015:
http://www.rand.org/pubs/monographs/MG720.html

Tedeschi, R. G., and L. G. Calhoun, "Post-Traumatic Growth: Conceptual Foundations and Empirical Evidence," *Psychological Inquiry*, Vol. 15, No. 1, 2004, pp. 1–18.

——— *Trauma and Transformation*, Thousand Oaks, Calif.: Sage, 1995.

——— "The Post-Traumatic Growth Inventory: Measuring the Positive Legacy of Trauma," *Journal of Traumatic Stress*, Vol. 9, 1996, pp. 455–471.

Tierney, M. J., and M. Lavelle, "An Investigation into Modification of Personality Hardiness in Staff Nurses," *Journal of Nursing Staff Development*, Vol. 13, 1997, pp. 212–217.

United States Air Force (USAF), *Comprehensive Airman Fitness,* Air Force Instruction 90-506, April 2, 2014, As of August 2014:
http://static.e-publishing.af.mil/production/1/saf_mr/publication/afi90-506/afi90-506.pdf

VIA Institute on Character, webpage, 2015. As of May 26, 2015:
http://viacharacter.org/HOME.aspx

Vogt, D. S., S. P. Proctor, D. W. King, L. A. King, and J. J. Vasterling, "Validation from Scales from the Deployment Risk and Resilience Inventory in a Sample of Operation Iraqi Freedom Veterans," *Assessment*, Vol. 15, 2008, pp. 391–403.

Wagnild, G. M., "A Review of the Resilience Scale," *Journal of Nursing Measurement*, Vol. 17, No. 2, 2009, pp. 105–113.

Wagnild, G. M., and H. M. Young, "Development and Psychometric Evaluation of the Resilience Scale," *Journal of Nursing Measurement*, Vol. 1, 1993, pp. 165–178.

Wald, J., S. Taylor, G. J. Asmundson, K. L. Jang, and J. Stapleton, *Literature Review of Concepts: Psychological Resiliency*, Vancouver, Canada: British Columbia University, 2006. As of April 9, 2011:
http://handle.dtic.mil/100.2/ADA472961

Wheaton, B., "Models for the Stress-Buffering Functions of Coping Resources," *Journal of Health and Social Behavior*, Vol. 26, No. 4, 1985, pp. 352–364.

Williams, R. B., E. D. Kirby, V. P. Williams, M. C. Hocking, and J. D. Lane, "Psychosocial Benefits of Three Formats of a Standardized Behavioral Stress Management Program," *Psychosomatic Medicine*, Vol. 68, 2006, pp. 816–823.

Williams, R. B., and V. P. Williams, "Adaptation and Implementation of an Evidence-Based Behavioral Medicine Program in Diverse Global Settings: The Williams LifeSkills Experience," *Translational Behavioral Medicine*, Vol. 1, No. 2, 2011, pp. 303–312.

Williams, V. P., S. L. Brenner, M. J. Helms, and R. B. Williams, "Coping Skills Training to Reduce Psychosocial Risk Factors for Medical Disorders: A Field Trial Evaluating Effectiveness in Multiple Worksites," *Journal of Occupational Health*, Vol. 51, 2009, pp. 437–442.

Yaskowich, K. M., *Post-Traumatic Growth in Children and Adolescents with Cancer*, dissertation submitted to the University of Calgary, Canada, 2002.

Yeung, D., and M. T. Martin, *Spiritual Fitness and Resilience: A Review of Relevant Constructs, Measures, and Links to Well-Being.* Santa Monica, Calif.: RAND Corporation, RR-100-AF, 2013. As of January 28, 2013:
http://www.rand.org/pubs/research_reports/RR100.html

Zach, S., et al., "The Benefits of a Graduated Training Program for Security Officers on Physical Performance in Stressful Situations," *International Journal of Stress Management*, Vol. 14, 2007, pp. 350–369.